J. G. McNulty

Interventional Radiology of the Gallbladder

Percutaneous Cholecystostomy

With 26 Figures

Springer-Verlag
Berlin Heidelberg New York
London Paris Tokyo
Hong Kong Barcelona

Prof. Dr. James G. McNulty
Diagnostic Radiology
University of Dublin
St. James's Hospital
P. O. Box 580
Dublin 8, Ireland

ISBN-13: 978-3-540-52905-7   e-ISBN-13: 978-3-642-75912-3
DOI: 10.1007/978-3-642-75912-3

Library of Congress Cataloging-in-Publication Data – McNulty, James G. – Interventional
radiology of the gallbladder : percutaneous cholecystostomy / James G. McNulty.   p.   cm.
Includes bibliographical references. ISBN 3-540-52905-5 (alk. paper). – ISBN 0-387-52905-5
(alk. paper) 1. Percutaneous cholecystostomy.   2. Cholelithasis – Surgery. I. Title. [DNLM:
1.   Cholecystostomy.   2.   Cholelithiasis   –   surgery.   3.   Drainage. W750 M478i]
RD546.M36   1990   617.5'56–dc20   DNLM/DLC

© Springer-Verlag Berlin Heidelberg 1990

The use of general descriptive names, registered names, trademarks, etc. in this publication does not imply,
even in the absence of a specific statement, that such names are exempt from the relevant protective laws and
regulations and therefore free for general use.

Product liability: The publisher can give no guarantee for information about drug dosage and application
thereof contained in this book. In every individual case the respective user must check its accuracy by
consulting other pharmaceutical literature.

Printing and bookbinding: Druckhaus Beltz, Hemsbach/Bergstr.
2121/3130-543210 - Printed on acid-free paper

To Professor Patrick G. Collins,
who made biliary surgery look easy
at The Charitable Infirmary,
Jervis Street, Dublin

Preface

Interventional Radiology has as its main goal the performance of surgical techniques using a percutaneous approach to simplify patient care. Percutaneous cholecystostomy now has many advocates; still, it is practised in comparatively few centers. Over many years it was used as a last resort at failed transhepatic cholangiography to provide images of the bile ducts in biliary obstruction.

Transhepatic cholecystostomy is reputed to be safer than transperitoneal puncture, since bile leaks do not enter the peritoneum. The advocates of percutaneous cholecystolithotomy, almost without exception, favour subcostal cholecystostomy and puncture of the fundus of the gallbladder. There is no evidence of bile peritonitis after successfully making a track to the gallbladder 18 F in diameter or larger for stone removal. After 1-7 days a postlithotomy drain is removed from the gallbladder and the patient is allowed home.

Transhepatic cholecystostomy for gallstone lysis, in contrast, requires only a 5-F track to the hepatic surface of the gallbladder. Loss of the gallbladder is not as great a fear with this technique as it is during dilatation of a subcostal track for cholecystolithotomy. During the latter procedure this may result in laparotomy to avoid bile peritonitis, while in the former, if the gallbladder is still visualised, the procedure may be recommenced immediately. Catheter dislodgement is a fear when prolonged catheterisation is considered. It can be avoided by using self-retaining catheters or by inserting several loops of catheter into the gallbladder. Delayed removal of the catheter from the gallbladder causes a fistula to form from the gallbladder to the skin, and, provided the cystic duct is patent and the biliary tract is unobstructed, the fistula closes and bile leaks are avoided.

Clear indications for percutaneous cholecystostomy have yet to be defined. It is advocated as an alternative to percutaneous transhepatic cholangiography for diagnosis and for temporary bile duct drainage. It has been most widely reported for gallbladder drainage in acute cholecystitis, where it competes with medical treatment alone and with emergency or delayed cholecystectomy. It has also been used for infusion of methyl tert butyl ether (MTBE) for accelerated stone dissolution after extracorporeal shock wave lithotripsy (ECSWL) in place of orally administered bile desaturating agents. It has been used for infusion of MTBE for dissolution of cholesterol gallstones, and this is probably its most important use at present since it is almost 100% successful in dissolving cholesterol stones, with minimum morbidity and no reported mortality. Stones of any volume and any size may be dissolved. Stone lysis time will decrease in the future with the use of mechanical rather than manual injections for stone perfusion.

Percutaneous cholecystostomy for gallstone removal uses a lateral or subcostal transperitoneal route to the gallbladder and track dilatation to 15-20 F for stone fragmentation and removal. Stone fragmentation is performed using electrohydraulic or ultrasonic lithotripsy with direct vision. Stone fragments are removed by mechanical means – with suction, a dormia basket or forceps. Gallbladder volume is kept small by continuous aspiration of fluid from the organ, and this makes stone fragment removal easier. Other potential uses of percutaneous cholecystostomy include gallbladder mucosal sclerosis and cystic duct obstruction.

Obstruction of the cystic duct causes a mucocoele if the gallbladder mucosa remains intact. Both gallbladder sclerosis and cystic duct obstruction are necessary for gallbladder exclusion, or "percutaneous cholecystectomy", in order to prevent gallstone recurrence. Current research indicates a gallstone recurrence rate of 10% per annum following therapy of small stones with the expensive oral bile-cholesterol-desaturating drugs. However, percutaneous cholecystostomy for gallbladder ablation is only a matter for theoretical discussion at present. Since in modern surgical practice not many patients have the operation of surgical cholecystostomy performed for acute cholecystitis, in most centres such cases will not be referred for percutaneous cholecystostomy. It must also be remembered that an acutely inflamed gallbladder is a friable organ without many contractile powers, and perforation of its wall occurs easily during manipulations within the lumen. In the elderly patient unfit for surgery, gallbladder drainage after endoscopic examination for biliary obstruction with ductal stone removal has a place in the treatment of acute cholecystitis, but it must be remembered that percutaneous cholecystostomy is more difficult when the gallbladder wall is diseased. Percutaneous cholecystostomy as a treatment for gallstones, whether by lysis, by stone fragment removal, after ECSWL, or by direct percutaneous lithotomy following electrohydraulic or ultrasonic lithotripsy, should ideally be performed only in a gallbladder with a normal mucosa and a normal wall as demonstrated by modern imaging techniques.

Attention should then be diverted to maintaining the gallbladder free of gallstones by diet and other means of desaturating bile cholesterol.

Ideally, interventional radiology of the gallbladder should be used to minimise patient discomfort, avoid unnecessary surgery, decrease morbidity and reduce convalescent time, and it should become a successful nonsurgical treatment for gallstones.

Dublin   James G. McNulty

Acknowledgement

This work would not have been possible without the assistance, stimulation and support of the staff of the Department of Medicine and Gastroenterology of Trinity College, Dublin University, at the Health Care Center, St. James's Hospital Dublin 8, and the University Department of Clinical Surgery at St. James's Hospital. I wish to thank Professor D. Weir and Dr. P.W.N. Keeling for referring patients and for their continuing support of the techniques of percutaneous cholecystostomy in the treatment of gallstones and Dr. Andrew Chua for his expert assistance with gallstone dissolution using methyl tert butyl ether. It was at the suggestion of Dr. Nap. Keeling, physician, gastroenterologist and expert endoscopist, that the author visited Dr. J. Thistle at the Mayo Clinic to study gallstone lysis techniques. At the Clinic Dr. Claire E. Bender demonstrated the methods of percutaneous cholecystostomy and she has continued to be most helpful with her knowledge and experience. Mr. John Brenna provided valuable information concerning storage, purification, and dispensing of MTB ether. I thank Professor T. Hennessy for his support, Dr. Luke Clancy, consulting physician, for referring patients with symptomatic gallstones for removal, and Drs. John Keating, Noreen Noonan and John Murphy and all the nursing staff for their assistance.

Contents

Introduction

The gallbladder is the final frontier for the interventional radiologist in the biliary tract and within the abdomen.

The normally functioning gallbladder is a very resilient organ, comparable to the urinary bladder. It has good muscular contractile properties and it is a safe organ to puncture percutaneously in the fasting patient using adequate analgesia, sedation and local anaesthesia. Subsequently, the organ may be catheterised over a guide wire and a catheter left in situ for periods ranging from hours to days or weeks. The percutaneous track to the gallbladder may be enlarged using coaxial dilators or a balloon dilator without ill effects. When the gallbladder wall is diseased, as in acute or chronic cholecystitis, it is easily perforated, so great care is necessary during intraluminal manipulations of guide wires and catheters.

In Western Europe and the United States the average life expectancy extends well over 70 years, and 22% of men and 33% of women may expect to get gallstones. Current opinion suggests that only a minority of gallstones give rise to symptoms and only less than 10% of individuals with gallstones require removal of the stones. Patients with symptomatic gallstones tend to be older and surgical mortality for elective cholecystectomy is 6.9% rising to 13.8% if the operation follows a bout of acute symptoms. Stones in the biliary ducts are also more common in the elderly, and there is added morbidity and mortality associated with biliary duct exploration in elderly patients. It is obvious, then, that nonsurgical methods of gallstone removal are a reasonable option for some patients. Stones in the bile ducts may be removed endoscopically following sphincterotomy with a much lower mortality than surgical exploration of the bile ducts.

Percutaneous cholecystostomy offers a new alternative to cholecystectomy for gallstones in the elderly and in patients considered unfit for surgery. Such nonsurgical methods for the treatment of gallstones which are effective in high-risk patients should obviously be offered to other patients with symptomatic gallstones as an attractive alternative to cholecystectomy. Following successful nonsurgical removal of gallstones, prevention of stone recurrence by dietary means and drug therapy is important, particularly in the younger patient, under the care of a gastroenterologist.

One of the most effective nonsurgical methods of treating gallstones in the gallbladder is dissolution of the stones by continuous infusions of the solvent methyl tert butyl ether (MTBE). This is effective only for cholesterol stones that are not calcified or that contain only flecks of calcium on the stone surface or have a calcified nidus. Since 60% or more of gallstones are composed of cholesterol, dissolution of these with MTBE should soon have wide application in all age-groups.

This technique, developed by Thistle and co-workers at the Mayo Clinic, is the easiest method available at present for the nonsurgical treatment of gallstones. Properly performed, it is an almost pain-free procedure which is without morbidity or mortality. We have found the technique to be very effective in patients of all ages. In contrast to other nonsurgical methods of gallstone removal, the equipment necessary for the procedure is widely available at minimal cost. As with other nonsurgical methods, the patient should have a functioning gallbladder, as demonstrated by oral cholecystography.

A Note of Warning Concerning Interventional Radiology of the Gallbladder: Percutaneous Cholecystostomy

Percutaneous cholecystostomy should be performed only by a radiologist experienced in percutaneous and interventional procedures. Treatment of gallstones or the gallbladder or biliary disease by this method requires the combined efforts of a physician gastroenterologist who is expert in endoscopic procedures, a competent biliary surgeon, adequate competent nursing staff, X-ray technologists and interested junior medical staff if the procedure is to be successful. Care of the patient before, during and after the interventional procedure is most important for patient safety and a successful outcome.

CHAPTER 1

The Anatomy of the Gallbladder

The gallbladder is a pear-shaped sac lying in a fossa on the visceral surface of the liver (Fig. 1.1). The size and shape of the organ vary with its physiological activity. Anatomically, it has three parts: fundus, body and neck. Between the neck and the body lies the infundibulum with an indefinite pouch (Hartmann's pouch) on its posteromedial surface.

The narrow neck is continuous with the cystic duct. The fundus is round and projects below the inferior margin of the liver, where it lies close to the anterior abdominal wall near the tip of the ninth costal cartilage. The body extends upwards and backwards from the fundus and lies in the line of the main boundary fissure, or *Hauptgrenzspalte* of Hjortsjo, which divides the physiological right and left lobes of the liver. The middle hepatic vein lies in this fissure. The posterior

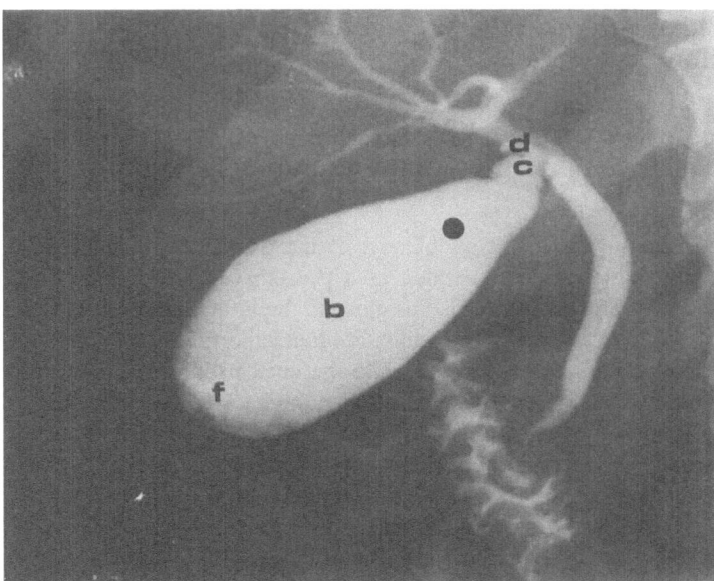

Fig. 1.1. The normal biliary tract (ERCP). *f*, fundus; *b*, body; *c*, neck of gallbladder; *d*, cystic duct; ●, ideal puncture site for percutaneous transhepatic cholecystostomy

surface of the organ is covered with peritoneum, while the anterior surface lies in contact with the visceral surface of the liver to which it is attached by areolar tissue and small vessels, mainly small veins. The gallbladder may lie with the liver substance or it may be suspended from the liver surface by a short mesentery [1].

The neck passes to the left to become continuous with the cystic duct, which joins the common hepatic duct to form the common bile duct. The posterior surface of the gallbladder is related to the first and second parts of the duodenum and the proximal transverse colon. Modern imaging has demonstrated many variations in the position of the gallbladder and many variations in the insertion of the cystic duct, into the common hepatic duct or into the right of left hepatic duct. An accessory cystic duct may join an intrahepatic duct in the right or left lobe of the liver. The gallbladder receives its blood supply from the cystic artery, which is a single vessel arising from the right hepatic artery in 80% of cases; in 20% of cases the cystic artery arises from the left hepatic artery or the superior mesenteric artery. Veins from the gallbladder enter the liver directly, or a main cystic vein joins the portal vein or its right main branch in the liver [3].

The gallbladder lymph vessels drain into lymph nodes along the common bile duct and into the coeliac nodes. Microscopically, the gallbladder has three layers. The outer serosa is the peritoneum covering the organ. It completely covers the fundus but only the posterior surface of the body and neck. The fibromuscular coat contains mainly dense fibroelastic tissue which is interlaced in every direction, and this is mixed with smooth muscle fibres which are mostly longitudinal. Muscle fibres also run transversely and obliquely in the wall. The internal or mucosal coat is mostly columnar cells with mucus glands. It is loosely connected with the fibromuscular layer.

Radiological Anatomy of the Gallbladder as Demonstrated by Ultrasound Examination

Prior to an examination of the gallbladder by ultrasound the patient should fast for 8 h. The gallbladder is demonstrated as a pear-shaped, echo-free structure with clearly defined walls. Its long axis lies close to the inferior surface of the liver and anterior to the right kidney. The fundus is often superficial and almost in contact with the abdominal wall anteriorly, while the neck usually lies in a deeper position. The fundus is more laterally placed than the neck. Gallbladder length is variable, but an anteroposterior diameter greater than 4 cm is considered pathologically enlarged. The fasting gallbladder wall is 3 mm thick. Hepatitis, heart failure ascites, hypoalbuminaemia, a contracted organ and cholecystitis are causes of wall thickening [4]. A pathologically dilated gallbladder has an AP diameter greater than 4 cm and is more round than pear-shaped.

In acute cholecystitis the wall is thickened, a sonolucent band is present in the wall, and low-level echoes are present in the most dependant portion of the gallbladder.

Radiological Anatomy of the Gallbladder as Demonstrated by Computed Tomography

Computed tomography of the gallbladder is carried out with the fasting patient in a supine position. The position of the organ in relationship to the right lobe of the liver is documented (Fig. 1.2).

The presence of calcium in a stone is documented without oral cholecystography. High-definition CT demonstrates stone nidus calcification, flecks of calcium in the wall of the larger gallstones or extensive rim calcification [2] (Fig. 1.3).

Sometimes an unexpected carcinoma is demonstrated using intravenous contrast medium, and focal thickening of the gallbladder wall may be evident with or without wall calcification in chronic cholecystitis.

CT scanning is seldom necessary for the diagnosis of mucocoele or acute cholecystitis. In the latter condition, a thickened wall, 1 cm or more, is visible outside the inner contour. This area is hypodense due to oedema of the gallbladder and increased vascularity. With contrast enhancement the inner wall can be demarcated from the outer layer of oedema. Local perforations show as hypodense zones. In emphysematous cholecystitis gas is present in the wall of the organ and in the lumen. In cases of mucocoele CT shows a dilated gallbladder, and an offending calculus in the neck may be present.

The CT scan of the gallbladder has an important function in assessing gallstone suitability for lysis with MTBE. In the fasting patient it may demonstrate a calcified wall in a large stone or flecks of calcium in the wall of the stone. A calcified wall of a gallstone is a contraindication to MTBE dissolution, but flecks of cal-

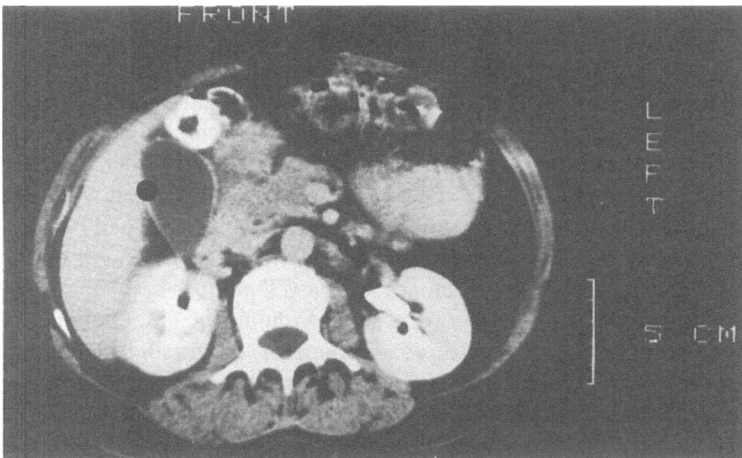

Fig. 1.2. CT scan showing relation of the gallbladder to the right lobe of the liver. Contrast medium is present in the colon and in the small intestine. An ideal puncture site in this patient is at the junction of the middle and upper third of the organ (●)

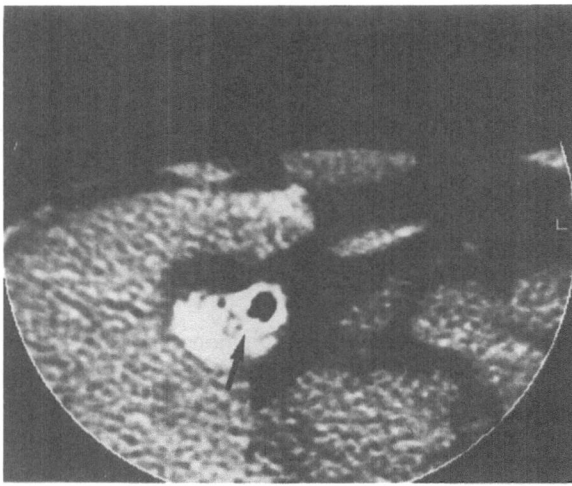

Fig. 1.3. CT scan showing calcified gallstones not suitable for dissolution (*arrow*), but suitable for cholecystolithotomy

cium are not. A nidus of calcium in a stone is also not a contraindication to dissolution with MTBE. A contracted gallbladder mucosa may mimic a calcified stone on CT.

Radiological Anatomy of the Gallbladder as Demonstrated by Oral Cholecystography

At oral cholecystography following the ingestion of an appropriate contrast agent, the gallbladder appears as a pear-shaped organ in the right upper quadrant of the abdomen. A single dose of contrast agent taken two successive days increases the density of contrast medium in the normally functioning gallbladder. A preliminary plain film is a poor indicator of calcified gallstones in comparison with high-definition CT but there are unsolved problems concerning stone density as measured by CT and the CT number of a gallstone above which the stone will not dissolve using MTBE. We have dissolved stones with a CT number of 140; however, the dissolution time is longer than that for a stone without calcium. Oral cholecystography is the best current method for determining that a normally functioning gallbladder is present. It is probably less accurate than ultrasound in diagnosing small gallstones. After a fatty meal the cystic duct and sometimes the common bile duct are demonstrated. This is not a reliable method of excluding calculi in the common bile duct.

An erect film of the gallbladder is important for demonstrating small floating gallstones, which are indicative of cholesterol stones.

Radiological Anatomy of the Gallbladder as Demonstrated by Direct Cholangiography

The gallbladder is opacified indirectly by direct cholangiography. Both percutaneous transhepatic cholangiography (PTHC) and ERCP easily demonstrate the gallbladder when the biliary tract is normal. In both these procedures the gallbladder fills retrogradely via the cystic duct. The gallbladder fills best at direct cholangiography when it is empty. Both ERCP and PTHC are very accurate methods of diagnosing gallstones when the gallbladder is adequately opacified. The gallbladder may also be selectively opacified by catheterisation of the cystic duct at endoscopic cholangiography.

Radiological Anatomy of the Gallbladder as Demonstrated by Percutaneous Cholecystostomy

Percutaneous direct injection of contrast medium into the gallbladder readily outlines the lumen. It is best if bile is aspirated completely from the gallbladder before injection of a dilute contrast medium. Even small gallstones are demonstrated. The cystic duct is opacified and the intrahepatic and extrahepatic bile

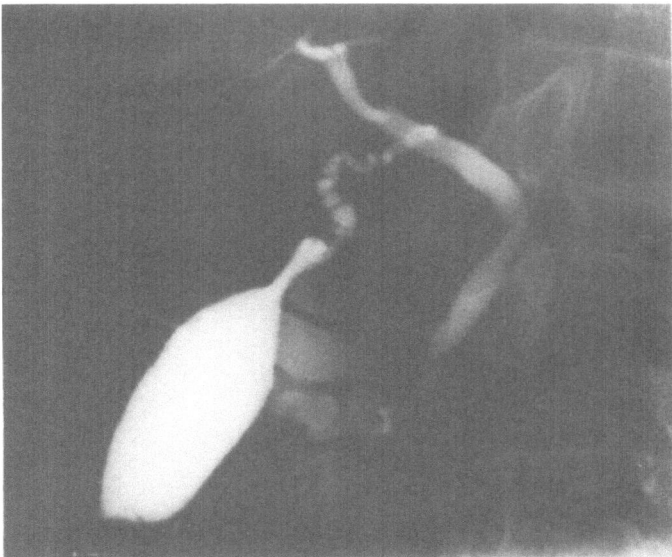

Fig. 1.4. Percutaneous transhepatic cholecystography showing a normal gallbladder, cystic duct and common bile duct

ducts are demonstrated to the duodenum (Fig. 1.4). It is important to make a record of the appearance of the bile ducts prior to stone-removal procedures to exclude bile duct calculi or other abnormalities.

References

1. Warren P, Kadir S, Dunnick RN (1988) Percutaneous cholecystostomy: anatomic considerations. Radiology 168:615–616
2. Middleton WD, Thorsen MK, Lawson TL, Folet WD (1987) False-positive CT diagnosis of gallstones due to thickening of the gallbladder wall. Am J Radiol 149: 941–944
3. Kahle W, Leonhardt H, Platzer W (1986) Color atlas and textbook of human anatomy, vol 2. 3rd revised edn. Thieme, Stuttgart
4. Bolondi L, Gandolfi L, Labo G (1984) Diagnostic ultrasound in gastroenterology. Piccin/Butterworths, Padova

CHAPTER 2

Percutaneous Cholecystostomy

Definition

Percutaneous cholecystostomy is the introduction of a catheter through the skin of the abdominal wall or axilla into the lumen of the gallbladder under ultrasonic or radiographic imaging so as to create a percutaneous fistula to the lumen of the gallbladder from the skin. The procedure is performed with the patient under local anaesthesia and with intravenous analgesia and sedation.

Indications

The indications for percutaneous cholecystostomy are:

1. Direct cholangiography
2. Biliary drainage
3. Gallstone dissolution
4. Gallbladder drainage after ECSWL
5. Gallbladder access for stone fragmentation and removal
6. Gallbladder drainage in acute cholecystitis or mucocoele

An *axillary* or *subcostal* approach to the gallbladder may be used. We favour the axillary route for all uses of percutaneous cholecystostomy unless a markedly distended gallbladder is visible and palpable in the right upper abdomen. While this monograph is concerned with the therapeutic uses of percutaneous cholecystostomy, direct puncture of the gallbladder may also be used for direct cholecystocholangiography when percutaneous transhepatic cholangiography (PTHC) and endoscopic retrograde cholangiopancreatography (ERCP) have failed to visualise the biliary ducts, particularly when these are not dilated.

In these circumstances percutaneous cholecystostomy is performed under ultrasonic control. The gallbladder is located with the ultrasound probe positioned anteriorly on the right hypochondrium, and a fine needle is introduced from the right mid-axillary line through the lower third of the right lobe of the liver to first indent and then puncture the right lateral wall of the gallbladder. The biliary tract is readily outlined by injecting a water-soluble contrast medium into the gallbladder (Fig. 2.1).

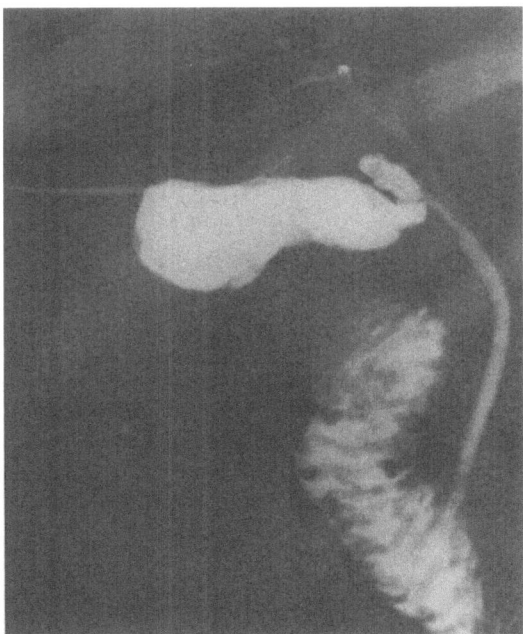

Fig. 2.1. Percutaneous cholecystostomy for direct cholangiography, demonstrating a normal biliary tract

We have found this procedure less useful when high obstruction of the biliary ducts is present.

Percutaneous cholecystostomy for drainage in acute gallbladder disease and for biliary drainage in extrahepatic biliary obstruction is considered later.

Contraindications

The only absolute contraindication to percutaneous cholecystostomy is an uncorrectable coagulation defect. In addition, the procedure should not be performed during advanced stages of pregnancy or when ascites is present. A porcelain gallbladder (calcification of the gallbladder wall), emphysematous cholecystitis or suspected gangrene of the gallbladder are also contraindications to this procedure.

A known primary gallbladder tumour is another contraindication, and obviously, percutaneous procedures are contraindicated in the bleeding disorders such as haemophilia and related diseases. Percutaneous cholecystostomy for the treatment of gallstones is contraindicated in the presence of a nonfunctioning gallbladder since in most cases this is an indication of gallbladder disease, and diseased gallbladders should be removed. We consider that gallbladder function is best assessed by oral cholecystography rather than ultrasound examination or HIDA scanning of the biliary tract.

Alternative Routes to the Gallbladder

The gallbladder may be catheterised via the cystic duct during endoscopic cholangiography. A guide wire is inserted during ERCP via the papilla of Vater into the common bile duct, with or without sphincterotomy. The wire is directed into the cystic duct and a nasobiliary catheter is passed over the guide wire into the gallbladder. Coiling of the wire and catheter within the lumen of the gallbladder is much more difficult than at percutaneous cholecystostomy. Positioning of the catheter around a stone for dissolution is also more difficult. This technique has been used to dissolve gallstones in the gallbladder with varying success [1, 2]. It may also be used for further treatment of the gallstone fragments after ECSWL.

Complications

Bile leakage is the most commonly reported complication of percutaneous cholecystostomy. This causes right upper quadrant pain and it is more common when the procedure is used to drain the obstructed biliary tract. When there is no biliary obstruction it is rare. Puncturing of the gallbladder via the liver for gallstone dissolution is rarely followed by bile leakage. Plugging of the exit from the liver at removal of the cholecystostomy catheter also reduces the chances of bile leakage. Loss of the gallbladder during track dilatation for cholecystolithotomy may cause extensive leakage of bile from the gallbladder after fundal puncture.

Diagnostic cholangiography via the gallbladder in acute disease and in extrahepatic biliary obstruction should be undertaken only after drainage and adequate decompression of the biliary tract for 24–48 h. This form of therapy is performed under adequate antibiotic cover in order to avoid septicaemia. *Vasovagal reactions* including nonfatal cardiac arrest have occurred during percutaneous cholecystostomy in patients with heart disease and recent myocardial infarction following mucocoele drainage. These reactions may be prevented by intravenous administration of atropine. As a precaution during percutaneous cholecystostomy continuous electrocardiography and blood pressure monitoring are essential.

Perforation of the wall of the gallbladder by a guide wire during catheter insertion is avoided by using a gentle technique of guide wire manipulation within the gallbladder. When a rigid wire is used to traverse a hard liver, then external fixation of the wire by an assistant is essential while the catheter is passed through the liver and into the gallbladder. If the gallbladder wall is perforated by a guide wire there may be loss of opacification of the gallbladder. This can be avoided by performing transhepatic cholecystography prior to guide wire insertion. A single perforation of the wall does not preclude proceeding with the catheterisation procedure.

A *Haematoma* may occur in the wall of the gallbladder due to incomplete insertion of the catheter/needle into the lumen and injection of contrast medium or and attempt to insert a guide wire. Both result in a local mucosal dissection of the wall of the gallbladder. If this happens the procedure should be postponed for a few days.

Puncture of other organs is rare with the transhepatic route of gallbladder puncture. During subcostal cholecystostomy the hepatic flexure of the colon may be traversed or punctured, and therefore great care is necessary when this route is used [3].

References

1. Ponchon T, Baround J, Mestas JL, Chayvialle JA (1988) Gallbladder lithotripsy: retrograde dissolution of fragments. Gastrointest Endosc 34:468–469
2. Foerster EC, Buhler H, Domschke W (1988) Direct dissolution of gallbladder stones. Lancet 2:954
3. Hruby W, Urgan M, Stackl W, Armbruster C, Marburger M (1989) Stone-bearing gallbladders: CT anatomy as the key to safe percutaneous lithotripsy. Radiology 173:385–387

CHAPTER 3

Preparation of the Patient
for Percutaneous Cholecystostomy

Percutaneous cholecystostomy may be performed as an emergency procedure for diagnosis and drainage of the gallbladder and/or biliary ducts or as a planned procedure for the nonsurgical treatment of gallstones. Emergency cholecystostomy is used for the treatment of acute cholecystitis, for mucocoele of the gallbladder and for drainage of the biliary system in extrahepatic biliary obstruction. Planned cholecystostomy is used for the primary treatment of gallstones as an alternative to cholecystectomy in patients who are unfit for surgery because of cardiac or other diseases and in other patients who opt for nonsurgical treatment when the alternatives are explained to them.

Emergency Cholecystostomy

Preparation of the often very ill patient for emergency percutaneous cholecystostomy should include hydration of the patient with intravenous fluids if dehydration is present. Cardiac failure requires treatment, particularly if the patient has dyspnoea. Rapid breathing by the patient is a contraindication, as there is a danger of causing a tear in the gallbladder wall during catheterisation.

Coagulation studies should show a normal profile, or abnormalities should be corrected before the procedure is performed. Patients receiving anticoagulant therapy require reversal of the coagulation defect prior to cholecystostomy. Pre-procedure antibiotics are necessary in patients who are at risk because of heart valve replacements or other cardiac defects which may lead to bacterial endocarditis.

The diagnosis of *acute cholecystitis* is made from clinical and laboratory findings, ultrasound of the gallbladder and HIDA scanning. Both ultrasound and HIDA scanning may have a low diagnostic accuracy in the hospitalised patient who is fasting or receiving parenteral nutrition, and percutaneous gallbladder puncture may be used for diagnosis of clinically suspected acute gallbladder disease as well as for drainage.

The diagnosis of *mucocoele of the gallbladder* is made by clinical examination and ultrasonography. Percutaneous cholecystostomy in acute cholecystitis or mucocoele of the gallbladder is performed under ultrasonic control. Percutaneous cholecystostomy for drainage of the biliary tract is used only when both endoscopic and percutaneous transhepatic drainage fail. The biliary tract in such cases is usually already opacified by the previous direct cholangiography, which also establishes the diagnosis of lower common bile duct obstruction.

It is of no value to drain the gallbladder when the obstruction lies above the common bile duct. These patients are often very ill because of cholangitis or liver failure secondary to biliary obstruction, and percutaneous gallbladder drainage is used for immediate relief of biliary obstruction. All patients with a history of heart disease are given 0.5 mg atrophine intramuscularly before percutaneous gallbladder puncture.

Planned Cholecystostomy

All forms of planned cholecystostomy are concerned with the treatment of gallstones by nonsurgical methods, including dissolution, direct removal, and removal of gallstone fragments after direct crushing with mechanical, ultrasonic or laser devices or ECSWL.

All patients should have a normally functioning gallbladder, and the oral cholecystogram is used to opacify the organ for visualisation. The patient continues to fast, and hydration is maintained by intravenous fluids.

Many methods of anaesthesia and analgesia have been advocated for percutaneous cholecystostomy [1]. These include intercostal nerve block, which is a very simple and effective technique but does not eliminate the pain of transhepatic catheter placement. Epidural anaesthesia is also an effective method of pain relief; for this, a well-trained anaesthetist is required, which increases the expense of the procedure and adds the complications of this form of anaesthesia.

We use a combination of pethidine hydrochloride and midazolam for pain elimination and sedation. Careful monitoring of respiratory and cardiac status is essential during the procedure. Midazolam also has a strong amnestic effect.

The elimination of the pain of percutaneous cholecystostomy has important results: The pain-free patient is more cooperative, the referring physician is more comfortable and there is less morbidity from the procedure [2].

References

1. Vogelzang RL, Nemcek AA (1988) Towards painless percutaneous biliary procedures: new strategies and alternatives. J Intervent Radiol 3:131–134
2. Lindemann SR, Tung G, Silverman SG, Mueller PR (1988) Percutaneous cholecystostomy. Semin Intervent Radiol 5:179–185

CHAPTER 4

Techniques and Equipment
for Percutaneous Cholecystostomy

The Fluoroscopy Room

A standard undercouch fluoroscopic tilting table with single-plane screening that is generally available in all radiology departments in hospitals and clinics is the only X-ray equipment necessary for percutaneous cholecystostomy. For all types of percutaneous cholecystostomy the patient lies supine on the fluoroscopy table with one or two pillows under the head. Two pillows may make the elderly of ill patient more comfortable. Both arms are placed at the patient's side, since the site for transhepatic or subcostal puncture of the gallbladder lies more anteriorly than the axillary puncture site used for PTHC. When percutaneous cholecystostomy is carried out for cholecystolithotomy the patient and X-ray table are covered in waterproof sterile surgical sheets which are available commercially. These are not necessary when percutaneous cholecystostomy is used for gallbladder or biliary drainage or access, or for gallbladder stone lysis. We find it best to remove the lead-rubber protection from the right side of the fluoroscopy table to prevent needle and guide-wire accidents during cholecystostomy catheter insertion [1]. Minimum fluoroscopy time screening is used, with the X-ray beam coned to the smallest area necessary for visualisation of the puncture track to the gallbladder during the manoeuvres necessary to catheterise the gallbladder. Using a transhepatic approach, the operator's hands should never lie within the X-ray beam. With the subcostal approach to the gallbladder, fluoroscopy should be strictly limited to assessing needle or dilator or catheter positions between manual manoeuvres.

A real-time ultrasound unit with 3.5 and 5.0 MHz probes should be available in the fluoroscopy room for gallbladder localisation when necessary. Ultrasound is essential for puncture of the gallbladder in acute cholecystitis and in mucocoele of the gallbladder.

Adequate space should be available for a sterile trolley and a drug trolley, and for lithotripsy equipment. The sterile trolley should contain:

Sterile gown and gloves
Local anaesthetic without adrenaline
Needles for local anaesthesia
Scalpel
Mosquito forceps
Containers of antiseptic and saline
Contrast medium, such as Ultravist 300
Syringes 10 ml, 20 ml, 30 ml
Sterile surgical sheets, sterile cover for X-ray control[1]
Sterile waterproof surgical sheets
Sterile gauze and cotton wool
Catheter needle for gallbladder puncture[2]
Guide wires[3]
Special pigtail catheter[4]
Set of coaxial dilators with an outer sheath[5]
Foley-type balloon catheter
Sheathed dormia baskets
Steerable catheters[6]
Suture materials
Biliary drainage set

Minimum personnel should include the radiologist, one assistant, one nurse and an X-ray technologist.

---

[1] 3M, USA, or Siemens-Elema, Solna, Sweden.
[2] Catheter/needles
   19-SWG, Surgimed, Denmark, 5.2-F
   Hellstern catheter needle, Angiomed, FRG
   Accustick catheter needle, Meditech, USA.
[3] Guide wires
   0.038 Lunderquist Ring Torque
   Amplatz Wire
   Radiofocus guide M, Terumo, Japan
   Lunderquist wire, Cook, Denmark.
[4] Special pigtail catheter 5-F
   a) 32 side holes in the loop Thistle catheter, Cook, Denmark
   b) Hellstern special pigtail catheter, Angiomed, FRG
   c) Self-retaining 7-F pigtail catheter with single-stick introducer trocar and retention suture van Sonnenberg catheter, Meditech, USA.
[5] Biliary coaxial dilators, Cook, Denmark
   Olbert balloon dilator, Meadox, UK.
[6] Steerable catheters, Cook, Denmark.

Protection of Patient and Staff During the Procedure

The use of an undercouch fluoroscopy unit results in the least amount of radiation to the patient, the operator and the assistants. Standard full-length lead aprons are worn by all personnel present in the fluoroscopy room during the procedure. These should have all-round body protection, because assistants present in the room spend a considerable amount of time with their backs to the fluoroscopy unit.

Neck protection is also used. Special hand protection is available with thin lead-impregnated rubber gloves which reduce radiation to the operator's hands.

In patients of reproductive age the pelvis is protected by lead covering of the table top beneath the patient (on the side of the X-ray source).

The total fluoroscopy time varies from 10–15 min for simple transhepatic catheterisation of the gallbladder to 30 min or longer for subcostal catheterisation and track dilatation for stone removal. Intermittent fluoroscopy during stone fragmentation and removal may add an additional 30 min to fluoroscopy time. We have not used biplane fluoroscopy for this procedure since we consider it mostly unnecessary, and it would increase the radiation dose considerably. Percutaneous cholecystostomy should not be performed during pregnancy.

Equipment for Gallbladder Puncture

There are two basic methods of gaining access to the gallbladder for percutaneous cholecystostomy. The most uncomplicated method is a "single-stick" technique in which a pigtail catheter is inserted over a trocar directly into the gallbladder. The van Sonnenberg Gallbladder Catheter (Meditech, USA) was developed for this purpose; it contains a retention suture which forms a loop that may be locked in position when the catheter is satisfactorily placed within the gallbladder (Fig. 4.1).

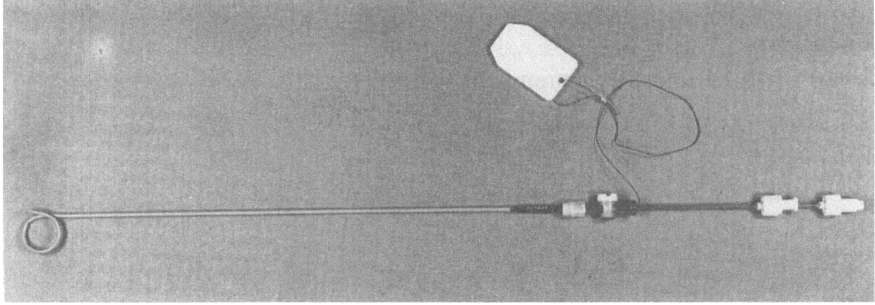

Fig. 4.1. Single-stick van Sonnenberg catheter and trocar loaded for insertion, Meditech, USA

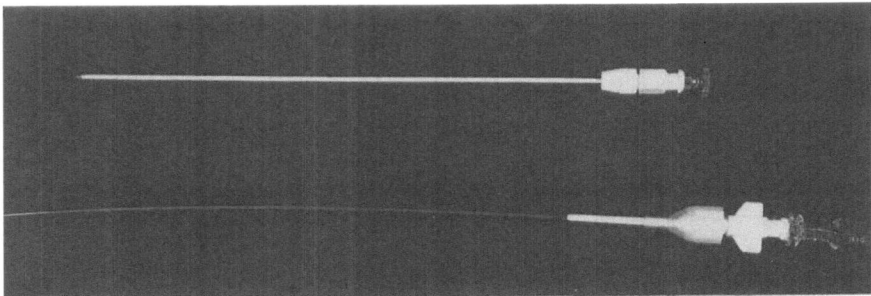

Fig. 4.2. Hellstern catheter needle, Angiomed, FRG *(below)* 19-SWG catheter needle *(above)*, Surgimed, Denmark

This catheter is very useful for drainage of the acute gallbladder in the short term. However, it is not possible to insert multiple loops of the catheter into the gallbladder by this method. The catheter is 30 cm in length, which we consider too short for safe positioning for gallstone lysis. It may also be inserted over a wire and coiled within the lumen. This leaves too little of the catheter outside the skin. We have also had difficulty in removing this catheter over a guide wire, as the guide is inclined to exit through a side hole when inserted prior to catheter removal.

The second method of gaining gallbladder access is by puncturing the organ with a catheter needle, removing the needle (Fig. 4.2), from which bile drips when it is correctly positioned, inserting a guide wire down the catheter into the lumen and coiling the guide wire within the gallbladder. The catheter introducer is removed and a special pigtail catheter is inserted over the wire into the gallbladder and coiled within the lumen. There are two catheters available for this procedure.[7] We have used both successfully in numerous patients for gallbladder stone dissolution (Fig. 4.3).

For gallbladder drainage in extrahepatic biliary obstruction we have used a 9-French pigtail catheter (Cook, Denmark) inserted over a guide wire transhepatically following puncture of the gallbladder with a 19-SWG catheter needle (Surgimed, Denmark). We have also used this catheter for subcostal drainage of gallbladder mucocoele and in extrahepatic biliary obstruction when the gallbladder is dilated and palpable anteriorly.

---

[7] 5-French Thistle Catheter, Cook, Denmark.
  5-French Hellstern Catheter, Angiomed, FRG.

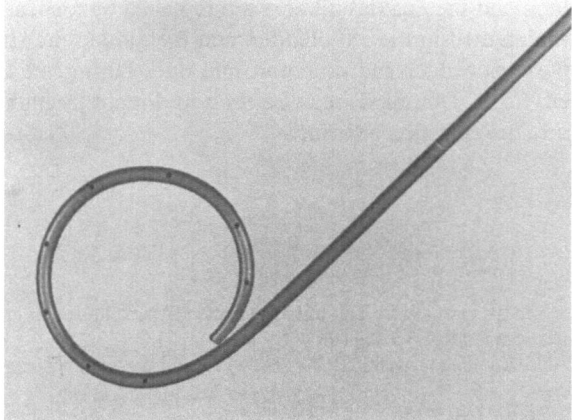

Fig. 4.3. Thistle pigtail catheter loop, Cook, Denmark; the Hellstern pigtail catheter is similar

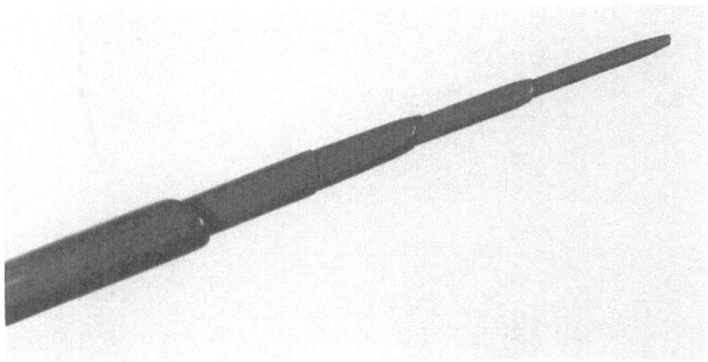

Fig. 4.4. Coaxial biliary dilators and sheath, Cook, Denmark

Gallbladder Dilator Systems for Stone Removal

There are two methods of dilating a track to the gallbladder. After percutaneous gallbladder catheterisation and irrigation for bile removal, either a balloon dilator (Olbert, Meadox, UK) is inserted over a guide wire to dilate a track to 12 mm (36-French) in diameter, or a series of coaxial Teflon dilators (Cook, Denmark) are inserted into the gallbladder over a guide wire [2, 3] (Fig. 4.4).

Both the balloon and the coaxial dilators are replaced by a sheath. At all times a guide wire is maintained in the gallbladder, and the guide wire should, if possible, lie within the cystic duct and common bile duct during track dilatation. A steerable catheter (Cook, Denmark) may be used to direct the guide wire into the cystic duct and into the common bile duct.

References

1. Bender CE, Williams HJ (1988) Technical aspects of percutaneous gallstone dissolution. Semin Intervent Radiol 5:186–194
2. Kellett MJ, Wickham JEA, Russell RCG (1988) Percutaneous cholecystolithotomy. Br Med J 296:453–455
3. Kerlan RK, LaBerge JM, Ring EJ (1985) Percutaneous cholecystolithotomy: preliminary experience. Radiology 157:653–656

CHAPTER 5

Percutaneous Transhepatic Catheterisation
of the Gallbladder
for Dissolution of Gallstones with MTBE

Percutaneous catheterisation of the gallbladder is easier when a route from the right axilla through the right lobe of the liver is chosen. Usually, only a short segment of the inferior part of the right lobe is traversed (Fig. 5.1). If the right lobe is slender inferiorly the area of liver traversed is minimal.

The presence of the liver track prevents bending of the catheter during its introduction over a guide wire into the gallbladder. Traversing the liver also helps to maintain the catheter in its original position within the gallbladder during dissolution therapy. The lateral approach to the gallbladder is easier than an anterior one and involves less radiation to the radiologist's hands, which are not working directly within the radiation beam when a conventional undercouch fluoroscopy unit is used. Puncture of the colon is also avoided. The aim is to puncture the body of the gallbladder in its middle third in the area where it is attached to the undersurface of the liver, and hence to avoid the peritoneal cavity. The track of the catheter should be parallel to the fluoroscopic table top.

A gallbladder on a mesentery is more difficult to puncture and it shifts medially to lie anterior to or just to the right of the lumbar spine when attempts are

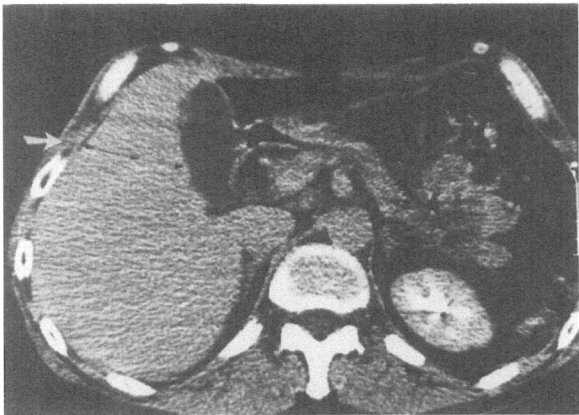

Fig. 5.1. CT scan of gallbladder. *Arrows* show the ideal track site through the right lobe of the liver to puncture the hepatic wall of the gallbladder at the junction of the upper and middle thirds

made to catheterise it. Puncture of this type of gallbladder is more painful, presumably because of traction on its mesentery. We have not encountered an ectopic, intrahepatic or pelvic gallbladder during this procedure.

Preliminary Studies

The diagnosis of gallstones today is made mostly by real-time ultrasound examination of the gallbladder. At this stage, the options for treatment of gallstones are described to the patient, along with the possible complications and morbidity of the various forms of therapy including surgery. When the patient chooses nonsurgical treatment or is unfit for surgery, further examinations are necessary to confirm that the gallstones are suitable for dissolution. Computed tomography of the gallbladder is performed in the fasting patient to rule out gallstone calcification; calcification of the wall of the stones excludes this form of therapy. However, flecks of calcium in the rim of the stones or a calcified nidus at the centre of the stones are not contraindications to dissolution therapy. (Fig. 5.2) [5, 6]. The CT scan also shows the relationship of the gallbladder to the right lobe of the liver and indicates the ideal site for gallbladder puncture.

If the stones are free of a calcified rim, an oral cholecystogram is performed to establish the presence of a functioning gallbladder, as indicated by good opacification of the organ. At this stage a date is fixed for stone dissolution.

The patient is admitted to hospital on the evening before treatment. A routine haematological examination including coagulation screening and liver function tests is performed. Further details of the technique are explained to the patient and written consent is obtained. A most important requirement for success of this procedure is calmness on the part of the patient and a positive mental attitude about the procedure. The latter can often be achieved by pointing out that he or she will be able to leave hospital within 3 days, minus the gallstones and without a large operative abdominal scar and with little or no discomfort. Such facts are more easily understood if the patient has a relative or friend who has had a cholecystectomy for gallstones.

Fig. 5.2. a CT scans showing calcified stone nidus in two gallstones. **b** Oral cholecystogram of same patient showing central calcification in the two gallstones. **c** Complete stone lysis at 5 h

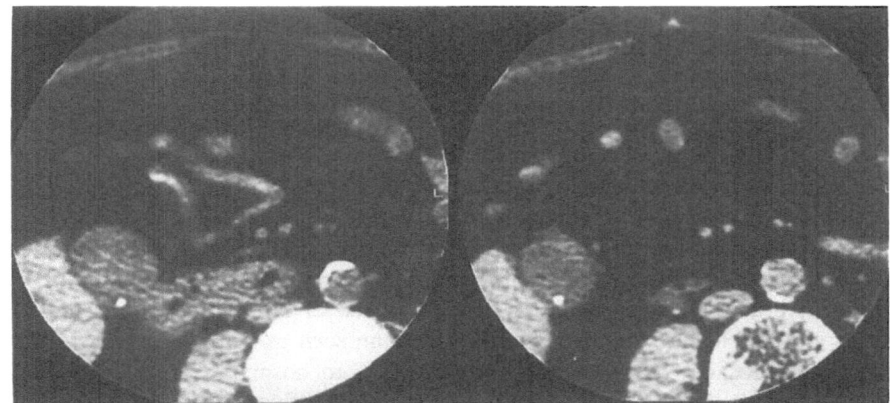

a

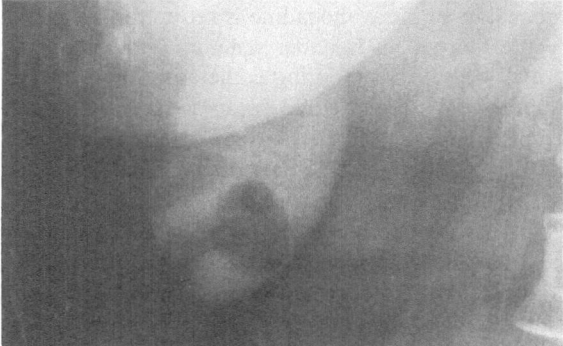

b

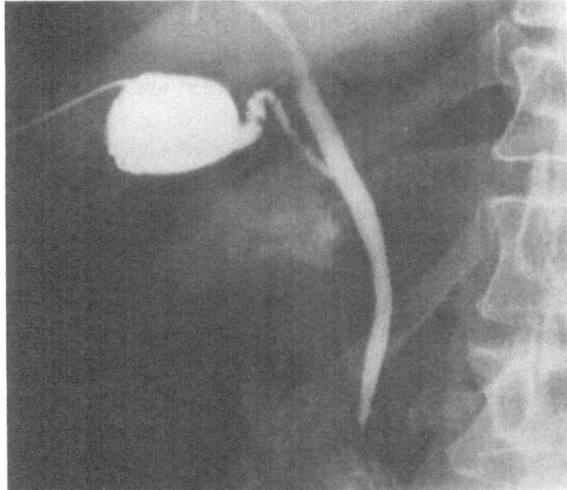

c

Technique of Percutaneous Transhepatic Cholecystostomy and Catheterisation of the Gallbladder

The procedure is carried out in the Radiology Department using a conventional fluoroscopy unit with an image intensifer and television monitoring. We have found that single-plane screening is adequate for gallbladder puncture in most patients and biplane fluoroscopy is seldom necessary.

The fasting gallbladder is a comparatively large surface area when compared with an intrahepatic biliary duct at PTHC, and there is seldom difficulty in puncturing the organ. For catheterisation of the gallbladder the organ is opacified by giving an oral cholecystographic contrast medium such as Biloptin or Telepaque in standard dosage on the evening of admission to hospital. The patient fasts overnight and has nothing to eat or drink until the procedure is completed. On the morning of the procedure an intravenous line is set up for hydration of the patient. During the procedure the patient is under sedation with adequate analgesia, and further analgesia may be necessary during catheterisation of the gallbladder. The patient lies in a supine position on the radiographic table with the head resting on a pillow and sufficient covering of the body to retain body heat. All clothing is removed from the upper abdomen. The area of the right side of the radiographic table is freed of all lead protection. An area in the right axilla is chosen as the site of skin puncture closest to the correct point in the lateral hepatic gallbladder wall. The site is located with fluoroscopy in the posterior-anterior plane and the skin of the right axilla is marked with a long forceps (Fig. 5.3 a). The exact site is drawn on the skin with a marker and the anterior-posterior depth is judged by consulting the CT scan of the gallbladder.

The site of skin puncture is usually a little anterior to the mid-axillary line. Next, the skin of the upper abdomen and lower chest and right axilla is cleaned with antiseptic solution and the chest and abdomen are covered with sterile towels.

Using an aseptic technique, the skin puncture site is infiltrated with local anaesthetic and the intercostal muscles and tissues are infiltrated down to the capsule of the liver. A small cross-shaped incision is made with a scalpel blade and with a mosquito forceps a track is made down to the capsule of the liver.

A catheter needle[1] is inserted through the incision towards the liver capsule and parallel to the table top and is directed under fluoroscopic control towards the site of puncture in the lateral wall of the gallbladder. Puncture of the gallbladder is easier when a site is chosen close to the neck of the organ in the upper third of the body, where there is more fixation of the gallbladder to the under surface of the liver (Fig. 5.3 b). When the catheter needle tip reaches the wall of the opacified gallbladder it indents the wall. Now a stab is made with the catheter needle into

---

[1] Needle 19. G x 190 mm; catheter 4.8 F x 170 mm (Surgimed, Denmark).

the lumen of the gallbladder. The movement is similar to that used for puncturing the femoral artery at arteriography. Simply pushing the catheter needle into the wall does not result in penetration into the lumen [1, 5].

The stylet of the catheter needle is now removed and black bile drips slowly from the catheter. Next, a semi-stiff guidewire[2] is passed through the catheter into the lumen of the gallbladder and the wire is coiled two or three times within the gallbladder. This is the critical point, and correct looping of the wire within the gallbladder lumen is essential for successful catheterisation (Fig. 5.3 c). It increases the stability of the transhepatic wire, and adequate looping of the wire aids looping of the drainage catheter. Next, the catheter introducer is removed over the wire and a 5-French pigtail catheter[3] with multiple side holes in the loop is inserted over the guide wire. It is passed rapidly through the liver into the gallbladder and coiled over the wire until three or four loops of the catheter lie within the gallbladder lumen (Fig. 5.3 d). Chilling of the pigtail catheter increases its rigidity and assists its passage through the liver and through the gallbladder wall.

Sometimes looping of the catheter over the coiled wire in the gallbladder is more difficult than described above. In this case it may help to slowly withdraw the wire one loop while advancing the catheter into the gallbladder and repeat this manoeuvre until three or four loops of the catheter lie within the lumen of the gallbladder.

Occasionally, the semi-stiff guide wire is not rigid enough to enable passage of the pigtail catheter over it without bending of the catheter and the wire between the skin surface and the gallbladder wall. This may be due to a hard liver, or it may be because the original track to the gallbladder does not traverse the liver owing to the configuration of the right lobe or because the gallbladder, although apparently in contact with the right lobe, is in fact lying free and has its own mesentery. When the semi-stiff wire fails as an introducer, a rigid Lunderquist wire[2] is used. The pigtail catheter is withdrawn and an attempt is made to pass the catheter introducer back into the gallbladder lumen and the semi-stiff wire is removed and replaced by the Lunderquist wire. Only the soft tip of this wire is coiled in the gallbladder and the pigtail catheter is inserted over it into the lumen of the gallbladder, using external fixation of the Lunderquist wire to prevent it from perforating the organ. When the pigtail catheter is one loop within the gallbladder the Lunderquist wire is removed and replaced by a semi-stiff guide wire which is coiled in the gallbladder. The pigtail catheter is now advanced over the looped guide wire as before.

When the gallbladder is not attached to the liver, puncture of the organ is more difficult. The catheter needle in this situation displaces the gallbladder medially, usually to a point anterior to or to the right of the upper lumbar spine. When pressure with the catheter needle no longer displaces the gallbladder the organ can be

---

[2] For guide wire types see list Chap. 4.
[3] 5-F Pigtail catheter with special side holes (Thistle, Cook, Denmark or Hellstern, Angiomed, FRG.

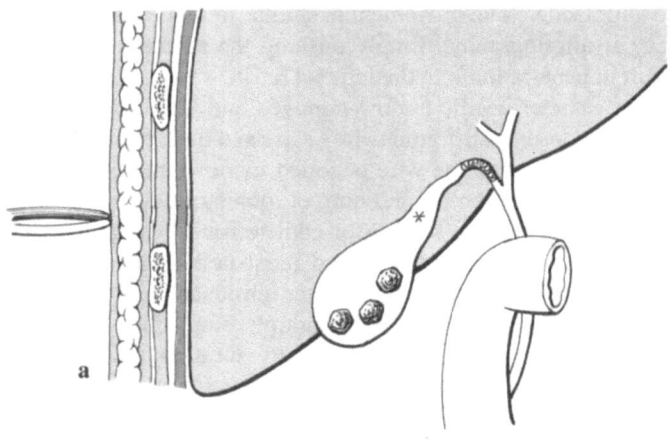

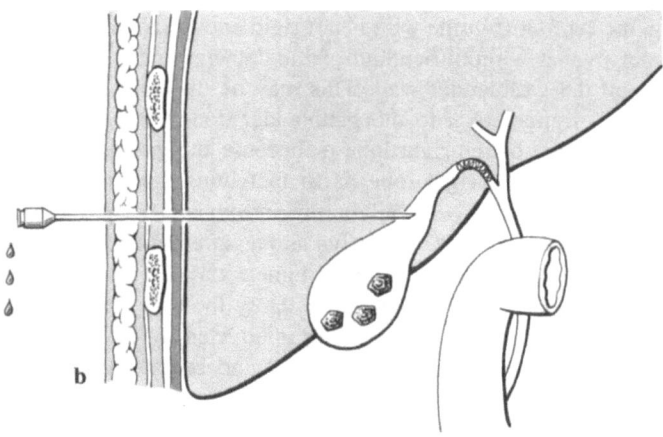

Fig. 5.3 a–d. Steps in gallbladder catheterisation. **a** Choosing the site of skin puncture in the right axilla. **b** Transhepatic puncture of the hepatic area of the gallbladder. **c** A guide wire is coiled within the lumen. **d** The special pigtail catheter is introduced through the liver over the wire into the lumen and coiled within the organ

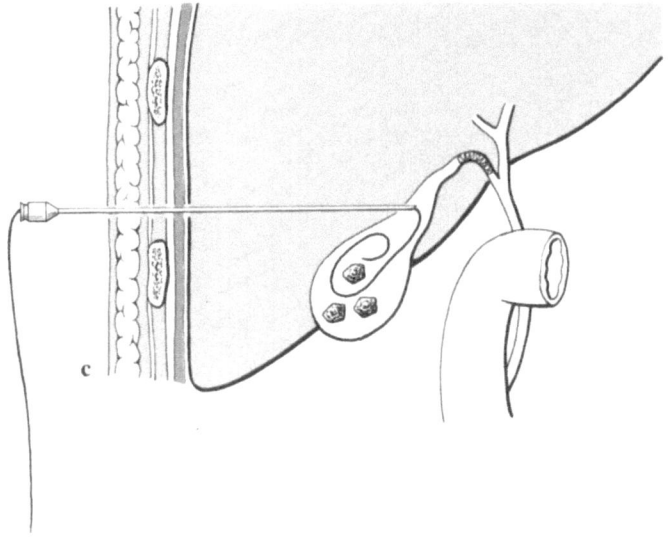

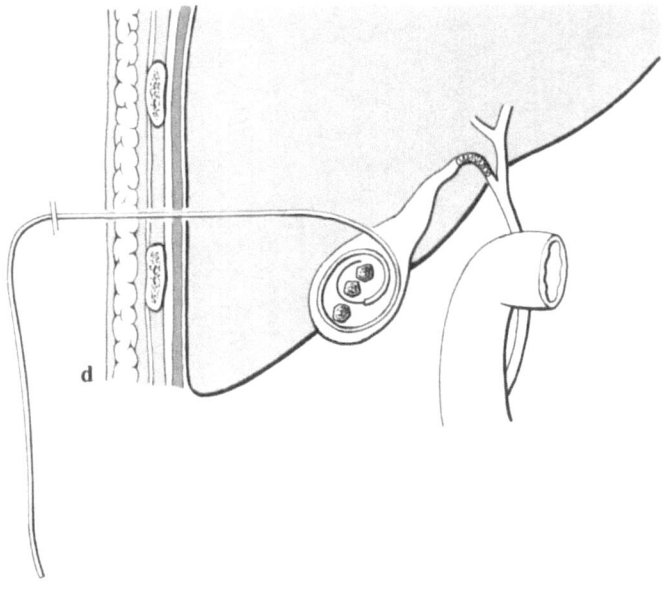

Fig. 5.4. a Oral cholecystogram showing a solitary large gallstone in an 84-year-old man with ischaemic heart disease. **b** Guide wire coiled in the gallbladder. **c** Catheter coiled around stone in the fundus. **d** Gallstone reduced in volume after 6 h of dissolution. **e** Gallstone totally dissolved; after 1 year the gallbladder remains stone free

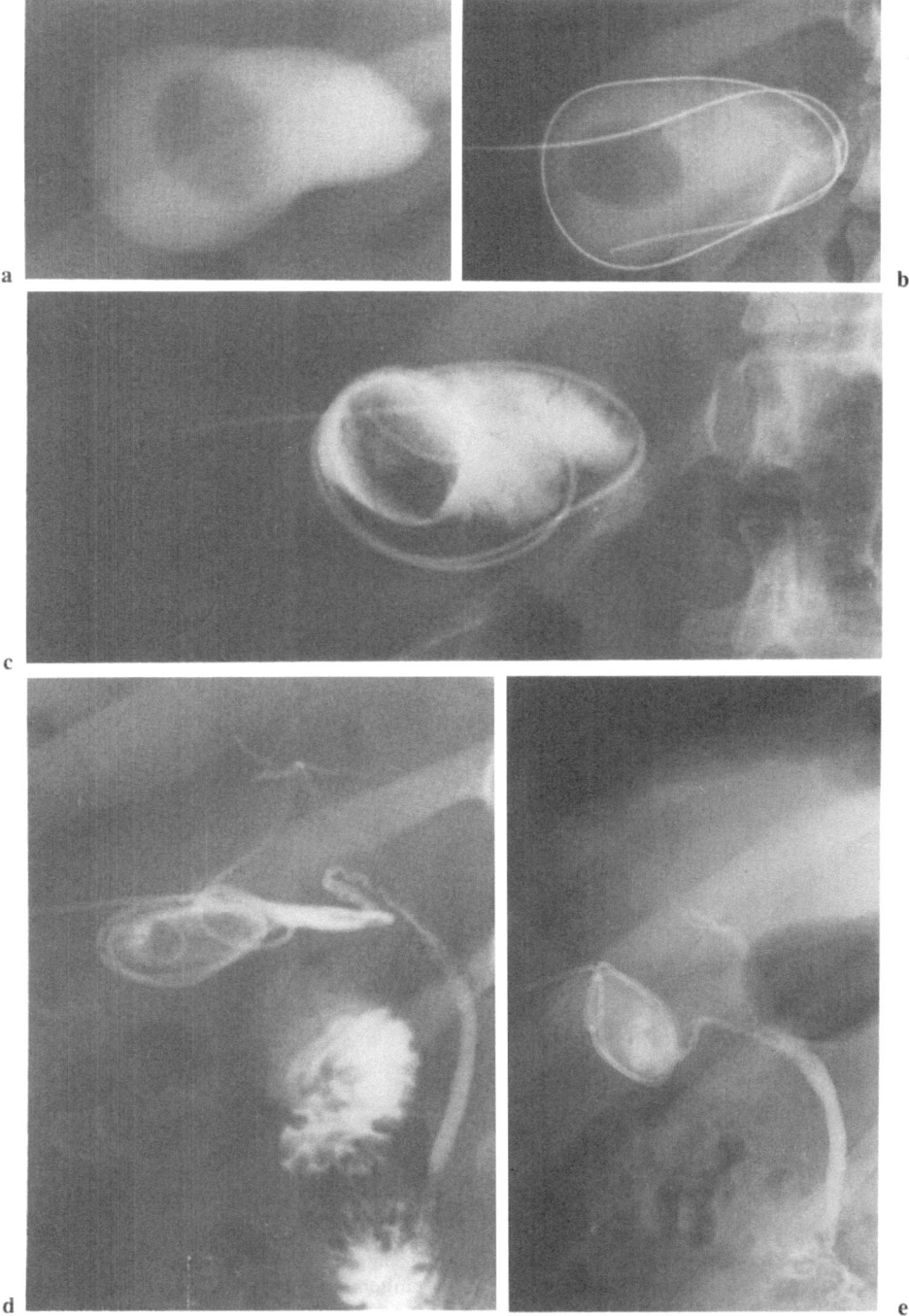

Fig. 5.5. a ERCP showing normal bile ducts and multiple gallstones in the gallbladder. **b** Percutaneous cholecystostomy. **c** Pigtail catheter being inserted over guide wire into the gallbladder. **d** Cholecystography after 3 h of dissolution. **e** Cholecystography after 7 h of dissolution; a single gallstone remains in the neck of the gallbladder. This was retrieved into the fundus using a loop of guide wire, and dissolution was complete after 8 h

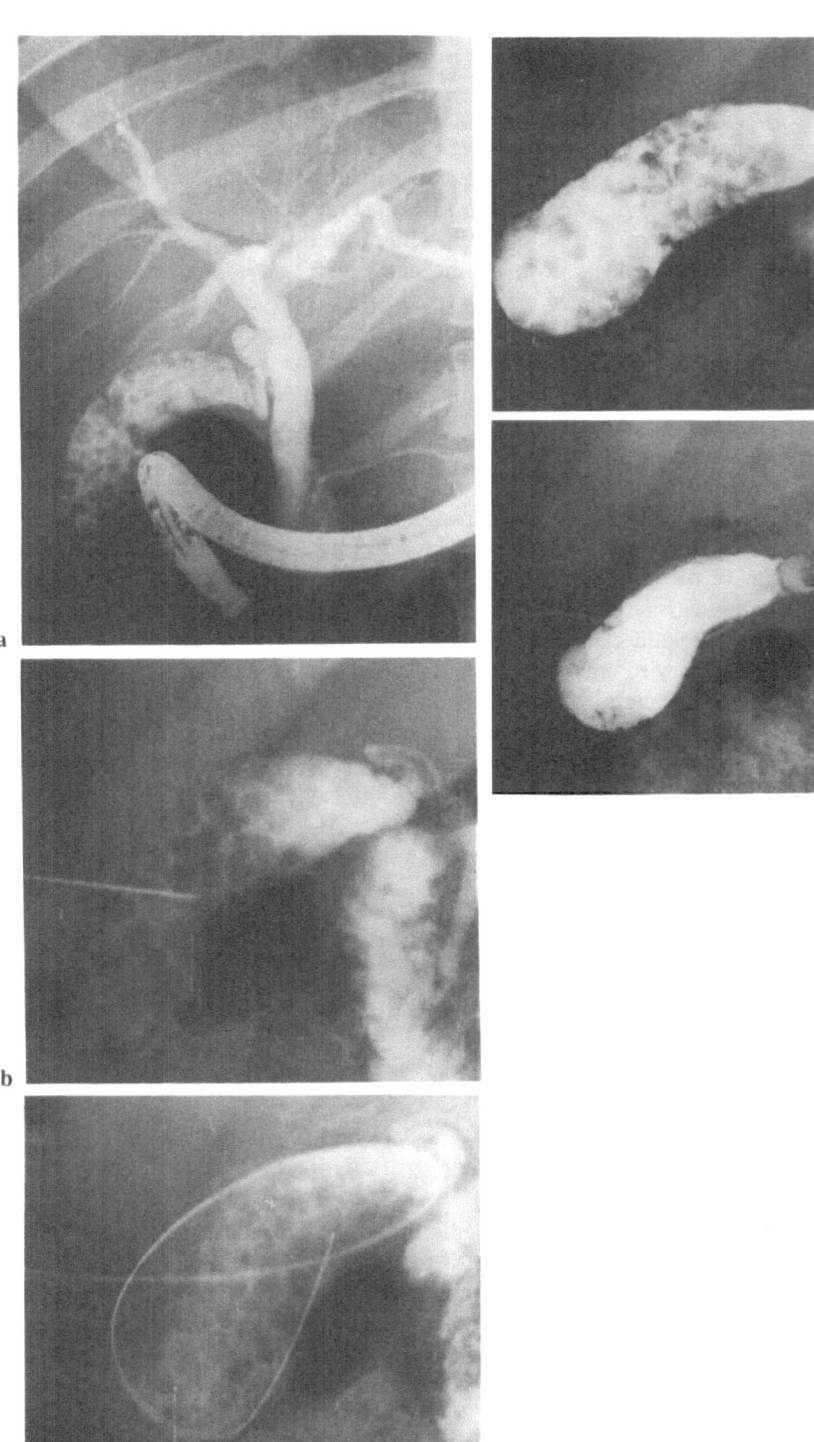

punctured successfully. When this attachment anomaly of the gallbladder is recognised, additional intravenous analgesia is given to alleviate pain caused by traction on the gallbladder mesentery which is attached to the liver.

After correct positioning of the pigtail catheter in the gallbladder all bile is aspirated from the organ and a water-soluble contrast medium is injected in order to determine the capacity of the gallbladder, demonstrate the number of gallstones present, outline the bile ducts down to the duodenum and demonstrate any bile duct stones. The pigtail catheter is now fixed to the skin of the axilla and connected to a closed drainage system. The patient is transferred to a special treatment room fitted with a special ventilation system with an extractor outlet close to the patient's bed, and the lower end of the bed is elevated 20°. Dissolution treatment is commenced immediately provided transhepatic catheterisation of the gallbladder has been uneventful.

If multiple small stones are present, the pigtail catheter distributes the MTBE through its multiple side holes and perfuses around the calculi, with the rapid stone dissolution. If a single large stone is present it is essential to move the stone into the fundus of the gallbladder and to position the pigtail around the stone before commencing dissolution (Fig. 5.4). Stone displacement and catheter manipulations with the gallbladder are carried out using a special wire.

It may be necessary to uncoil the catheter loops to achieve fundal stone placement or to move the pigtail catheter around within the gallbladder. The stone movement is achieved by pushing it with a straight or an angled guide wire. The catheter placement around the stone is achieved by first positioning the guide wire around the stone and then coiling the pigtail of the catheter over the wire around the stone (Fig. 5.5).

Complications

Complications are uncommon when a careful technique is used [2, 3, 6]. We encountered the following complications during the process of learning the technique.

Injection of the Wall of the Gallbladder

As mentioned earlier, if the catheter needle tip is not introduced far enough into the lumen, or if it is introduced too far, it may perforate the opposite wall. Bile may drip from the catheter but injected contrast medium will outline only part of the gallbladder wall. The outline may resemble the gallbladder, but of course the gallstones are not visualised. When this occurs the catheter must be withdrawn and another attempt made to puncture the lumen successfully can then be continued.

Perforation of the Gallbladder with the Guide Wire

This may occur during attempts at coiling the wire. It is of no significance when it is recognised and the wire is withdrawn back into the gallbladder. It is usually necessary to withdraw the wire completely and begin again with catheter needle puncture of the gallbladder. In some patients perforation of the gallbladder with the wire results in loss of gallbladder opacification, or the opacification is too poor for visualisation of the organ by fluoroscopy. When this happens, ultrasound may be used to visualise the gallbladder and indentation of the gallbladder wall by the catheter needle tip is easily visualised before puncture of the lumen. After successful puncture the procedure is continued as above. In order to prevent complete loss of gallbladder opacification when the wall is perforated by the guide wire, the gallbladder may be densely opacified by injection of contrast medium when the gallbladder is initially punctured with the catheter needle.

A single perforation of the gallbladder closes off almost immediately after the wire is withdrawn and is not an indication for termination of the procedure. When it is followed by successful catheterisation of the gallbladder, dissolution therapy can be commenced after a delay of 4 h. Before treatment is begun, contrast medium is injected into the gallbladder to confirm that there are no signs of leakage from the perforation site.

If there is a small leak of contrast medium from the area of the gallbladder wall punctured by the wire the dissolution is postponed for 24 h, after which interval the gallbladder is again outlined with contrast medium; it is very rare to still find leakage from the puncture site at this point.

Other complications reported in the literature have been covered in Chap. 2.

Cholesterol Gallstone Dissolution with MTBE

Properties of the Solvent Methyl Tert Butyl Ether

It is known that cholesterol gallstones dissolve rapidly in diethyl ether. The ether vapourises at 34.5 °C. Methyl tert butyl ether (MTBE) has physical properties almost identical to those of diethyl ether but its boiling point is higher (55.2 °C). It thus remains a liquid at body temperatures. The physical properties of MTBE are:

Formula	–	$C_5 H_{12} O$
Mol. wt.	–	88.14
Specific gravity	–	0.741
Boiling point	–	55.2 °C
Ignition temperature	–	224 °C
Viscosity	–	0.27
Oral toxicity	–	4000mg/kg (mouse)

MTBE dissolves cholesterol gallstones rapidly in vitro. In vivo studies in dogs in whom human cholesterol gallstones were implanted surgically showed that the stones dissolved rapidly following instillation of MTBE via a surgically implanted gallbladder catheter. Histology of the gallbladder subsequently showed no evidence of gallbladder injury from the MTBE.

MTBE is a flammable solvent with explosive properties. It requires careful storage in a flameproof cabinet. It is kept in glass containers which are tightly capped or in metal cans. MTBE is a strong solvent which affects many plastics such as those used in disposable syringes and specimen containers. Plastic syringes or bottles cannot be used to house this solvent. It must be injected using glass syringes which do not have rubber stoppers, as rubber is also dissolved by MTBE. MTBE does not dissolve the pigtail catheter, which is manufactured from low-density polyethylene.

MTBE is used as an octane enhancer in petrol. It is 97% pure. Distillation and microfiltration are used to sterilise the solvent prior to instillation into the gallbladder.

MTBE floats on bile, while cholesterol stones sink, and adequate contact of the solvent with the stone requires continuous mixing by injection and withdrawl through the pigtail catheter. Stone-solvent contact is a critical factor in determining the rate of gallstone dissolution. Ideally, an infusion pump which allows rapid injection of MTBE followed by slow aspiration would shorten dissolution time.

When used clinically, great care is necessary to prevent accidents with this potentially explosive solvent. After gallstone treatment the ether/bile/cholesterol mixture should be disposed of as a toxic-waste product.

The Technique of Gallstone Dissolution

The treatment room must at all times have good ventilation. An extractor for removal of the ether vapour is installed, situated close to the patient's abdomen and to the doctor or nurse carrying out the dissolution. A number of glass syringes containing increasing volumes of MTBE are prepared and stored in a rack in the treatment room. Infusion of solvent is begun with injection and aspiration of 2 ml continuously for 30 min; this is increased to infusion and aspiration of 3 ml for 30 min, with frequent changes of the syringe as the MTBE becomes saturated with cholesterol. The amount of MTBE is increased at intervals until 10-ml volumes are being continually infused and aspirated.

At intervals, a staff member visits the treatment room and tests by sniffing to see if the patient is expelling MTBE from the lungs. Treatment sessions of 3 h twice daily are undertaken until all of the calculi are dissolved as evidenced by absence of cholesterol from the aspirate. If ether is detected in the patient's breath the session is terminated for 3–4 h. Most gallstones are dissolved with 6–9 h of MTBE infusion. At the first injection of 2 ml MTBE right upper quadrant pain may be felt by the patient. If this happens non-narcotic analgesics are given and continuous light sedation is maintained throughout the stone-dissolution periods.

When the stones are clinically dissolved, the patient is returned to the Radiology Department and the gallbladder is opacified via the pigtail catheter using dilute contast agent to confirm total stone dissolution. In any event, if the catheter is in situ in the gallbladder overnight its position in the lumen should be confirmed the following morning before dissolution is again commenced. When the opacified gallbladder shows no further stones MTBE infusions are continued for a further 3 h and the patient is again referred back to the Radiology Department for removal of the catheter from the gallbladder. It is most important during the procedure to keep the patient fully informed of the progress of the stone dissolution, and an optimistic outlook towards the patient's progress on the part of the medical and nursing staff will ensure continued co-operation.

In some patients nausea occurs as treatment progresses and this is treated symptomatically. We have noted on sequential contrast studies of the gallbladder that some spasm or contraction of the gallbladder occurs, and this may be associated with pain in the upper abdomen. It is best if the patient does not eat during the period of dissolution treatment. Hydration of the patient is maintained by intravenous fluids. Some of our patients had food, however, by accident or intrigue, during intervals between treatments. This has caused gallbladder pain in some cases, but in others food has had no ill effects.

During intervals between treatments the catheter is connected to a closed drainage system, and the patient is informed that it is very much in his or her interest to see that the catheter does not become dislodged. Multiple small stones dissolve rapidly in 3 or 4 h with MTBE therapy, while a large solitary cholesterol stone may take 6 or more hours to break into fragments or to fissure. Once the stone fissures or fragments, dissolution is rapid. Several large stones may also dissolve rapidly with 4–5 h of dissolution therapy (Fig. 5.6–5.8).

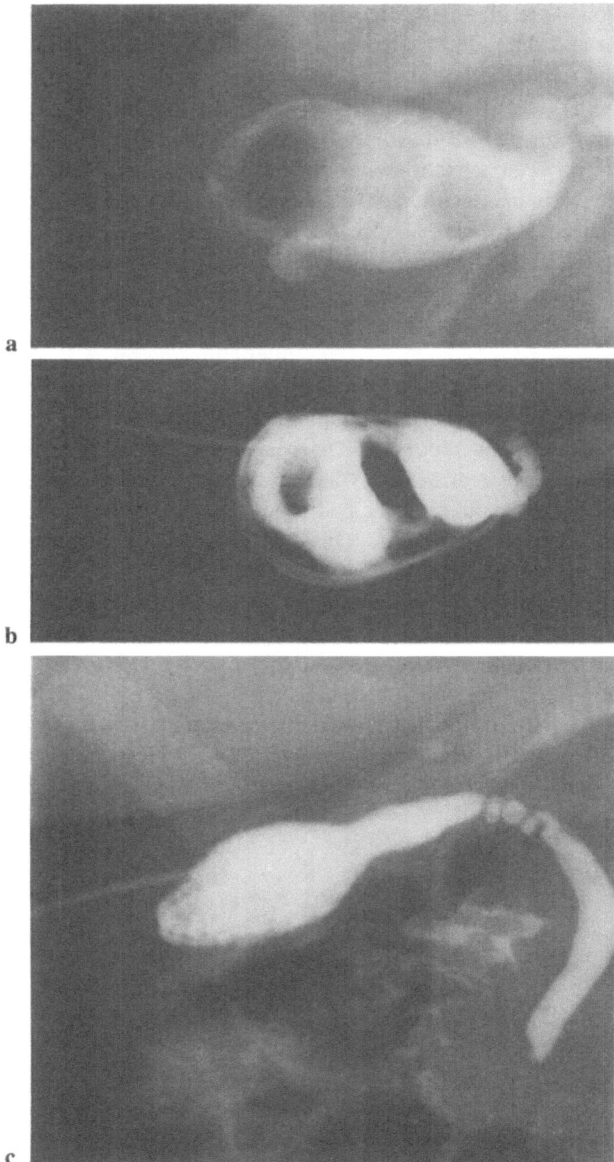

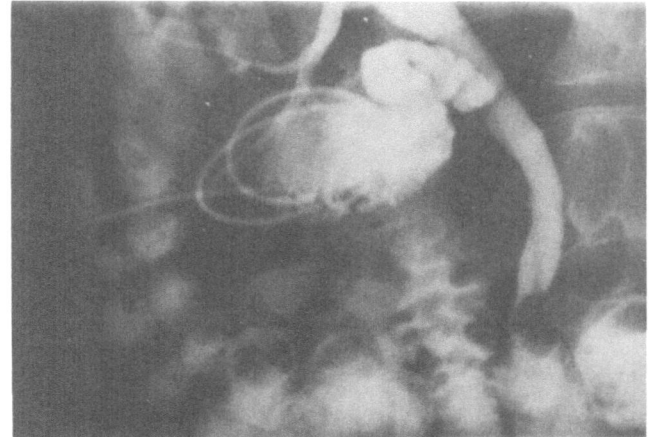

d

Fig. 5.6. a Cholecystogram showing multiple stones in the gallbladder. **b** Cholecystography at 6 h showing stone fragmentation and partial dissolution. **c** Cholecystography at 12 h showing complete stone lysis and no contrast medium passing from the common bile duct into the duodenum. **d** Repeat percutaneous cholecystocholangiography after saline irrigation of the gallbladder and bile ducts, during which the patient complained of severe abdominal pain. A calculus is impacted at the papilla. This was immediately removed by endoscopic sphincterotomy. The patient remains stone free after 13 months

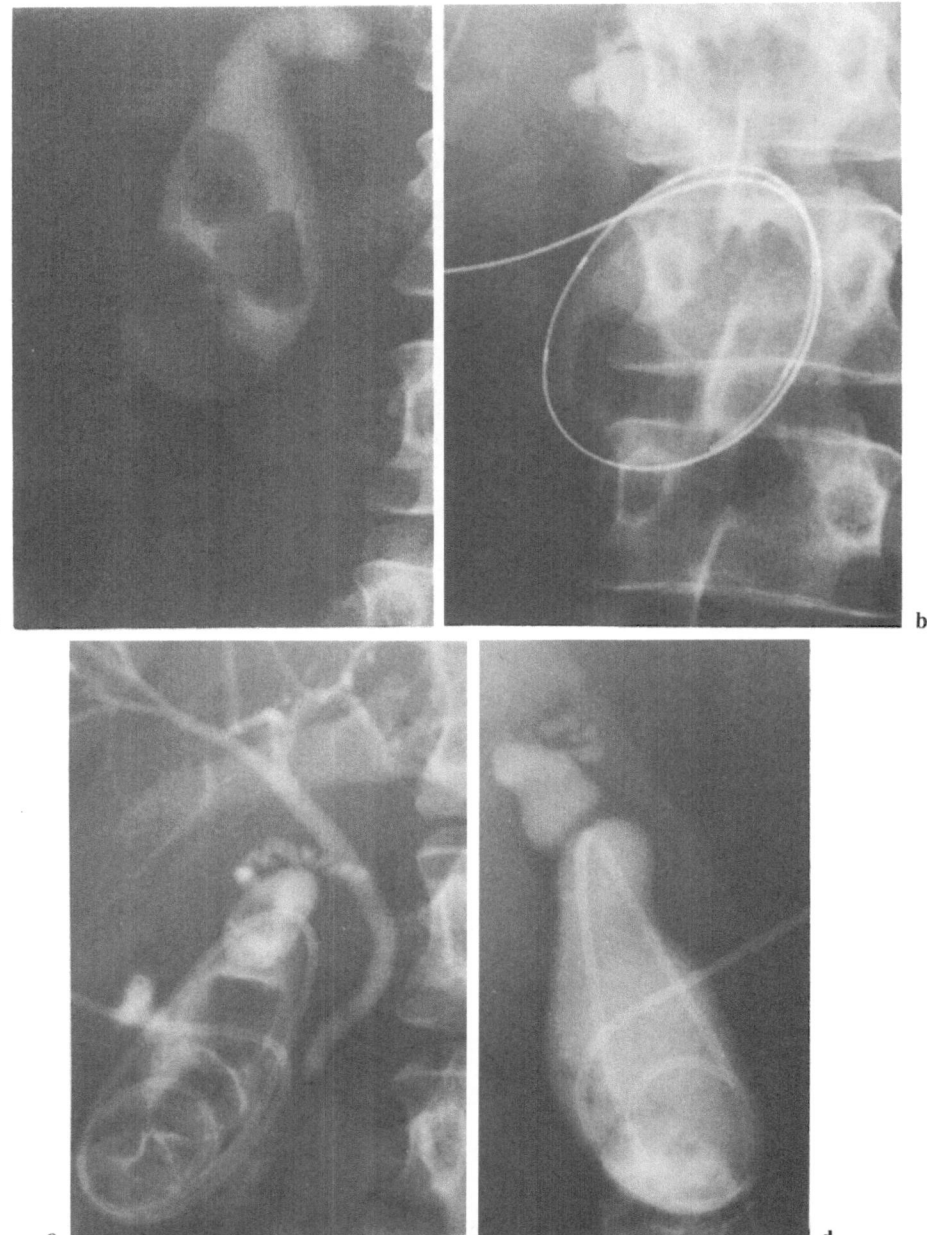

Fig. 5.7. a Oral cholecystogram showing five large gallstones. **b** Guide wire coiled within the gallbladder. The latter has a mesentery and now lies partly over the lumbar spine. **c** After 6 h dissolution. **d** After 12 h dissolution, the gallbladder and bile ducts are stone free: Prone view of gallbladder showing debris

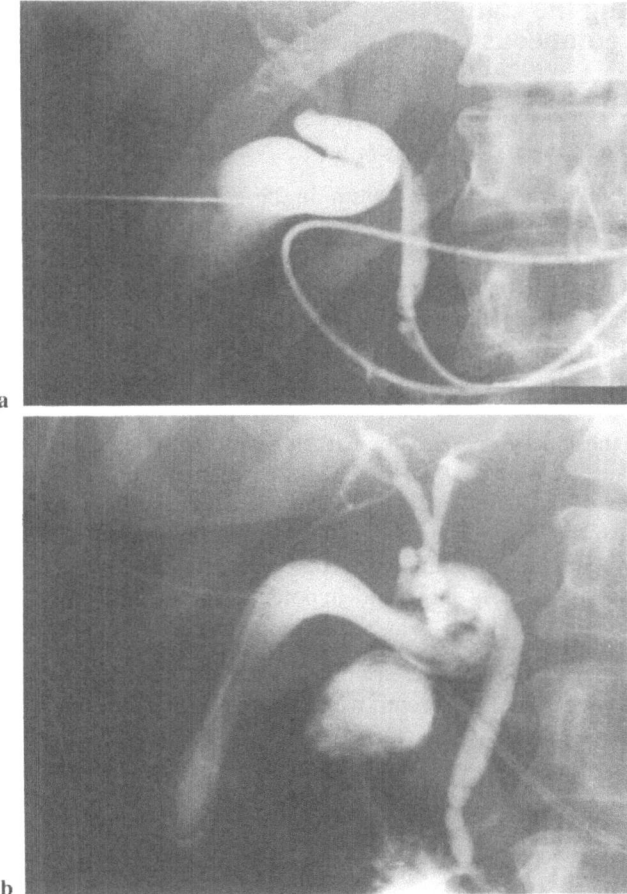

Fig. 5.8. a Cholangiogram by injection of contrast medium into a nasobiliary catheter demonstrated multiple gallstones and normal bile ducts. Percutaneous catheter/needle is inserted into the gallbladder. **b** Cholecystogram via the cholecystostomy catheter shows complete stone dissolution at 3 h

Repositioning the Catheter
During Percutaneous Cholecystostomy for Dissolution Therapy

There are two reasons why it may be necessary to reposition the catheter during percutaneous dissolution of gallstones:

a) The gallbladder may have a septum in the body, with stones present in both compartments of the organ. After dissolution of gallstones in one compartment it is necessary to adjust the position of the catheter pigtail loop and to place it in the second compartment so that it bathes the stones in that area with the MTBE.

b) During an overnight interval between sessions of dissolution the catheter may become partly dislodged from the lumen of the gallbladder, and predissolution cholecystography may show that there is a leak of contrast medium from one of the side holes in the pigtail loop. This is most likely to occur when the gallbladder has a mesentery or when the catheter is not inserted transhepatically via the axilla because of a narrow anterior-posterior diameter of the right lobe of the liver in the area of the catheter track. It may also occur, particularly in the elderly patient, as a result of traction on the catheter from the outside, so fixation of the catheter to the abdominal wall must be secure. Occasionally, when the gallbladder is long and narrow or very large and hypotonic, the catheter may become dislodged because not enough of it was placed in the lumen originally.

In these instances the catheter is repositioned in the lumen using the guide wire. We have found that the Terumo wire is best for this purpose (Fig. 5.9 a–e).

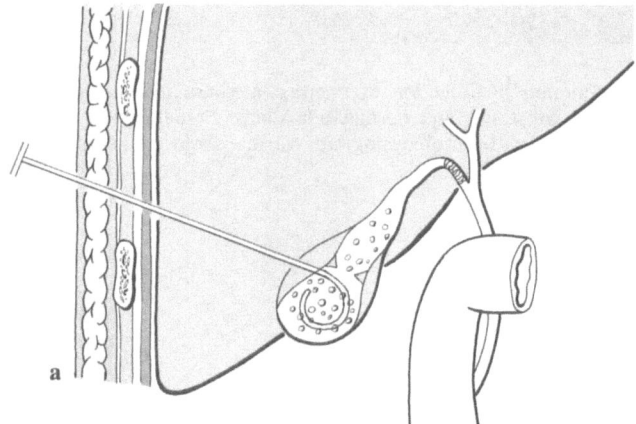

Fig. 5.9. a–e. Changing the catheter position within the gallbladder. **a** Catheter in the fundus of the gallbladder or lower compartment of the gallbladder. **b** The catheter is withdrawn over a guide wire until the pigtail is straight (**c**)

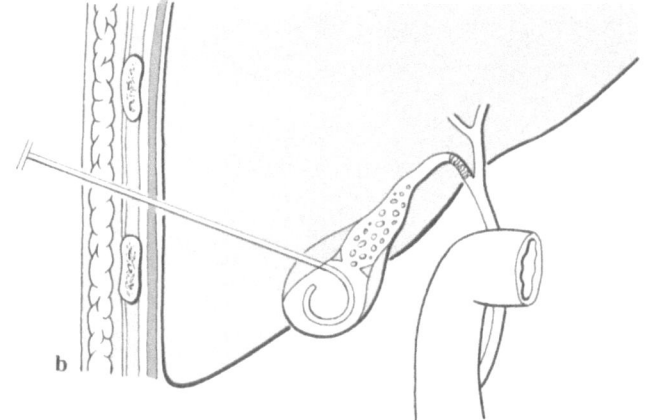

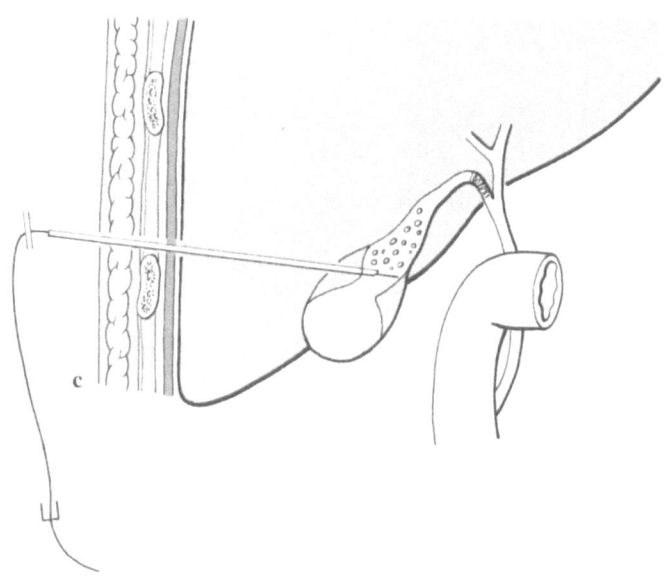

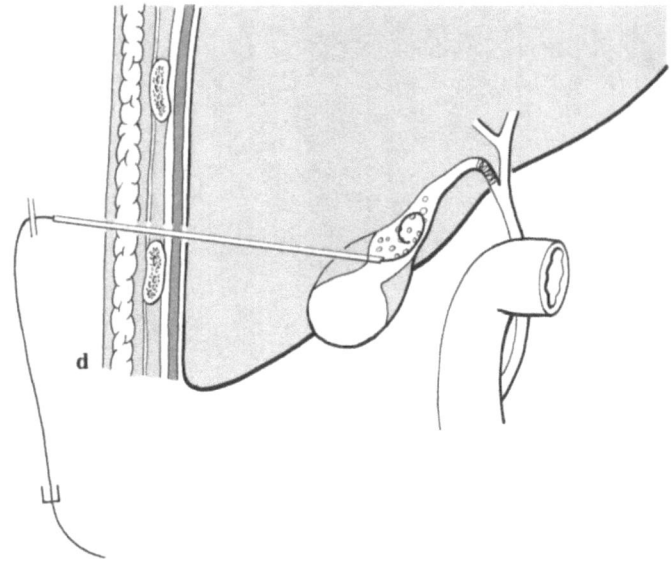

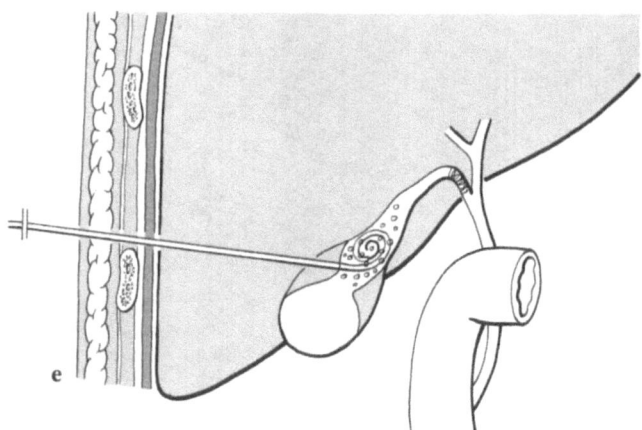

Fig. 5.9. d The wire is pushed into the neck or upper compartment and the catheter is reintroduced over the wire. **e** Catheter is pushed over the wire into the fundus and coiled

Repositioning the Catheter Around Gallstones

The guide wire is inserted into the catheter until its tip lies free in the lumen. The catheter loops within the lumen are uncoiled, care being taken not to remove the catheter totally from the lumen. The guide wire is then positioned into the area of the gallbladder where the stones lie and it is looped in this position. The catheter is now advanced over the wire into the required position and the wire is removed.

Repositioning the Partly Dislodged Catheter

The guide wire is carefully inserted into the catheter until its tip reaches the lumen of the gallbladder. The catheter is fixed at the skin by an assistant to prevent it being dislodged further by the guide wire. The wire is now carefully inserted into the gallbladder lumen and coiled within the lumen. The catheter is pushed over the wire into the gallbladder and looped several times within the lumen. The wire is removed, and dissolution is recommenced after an interval of 2–4 h, and after it has been ascertained by means of predissolution cholecystography that there is no leakage.

Manipulation of a Stone from the Neck into the Body of the Gallbladder

When a stone becomes lodged in the neck of the gallbladder during gallstone lysis or fragmentation it is necessary to manipulate it back into the lumen of the body of the gallbladder. A guide wire is inserted into the gallbladder lumen via the in situ catheter. A loop of the wire or wire covered by catheter is pushed into the gallbladder neck to surround the stone, and withdrawl of the loop engages the stone, replacing it into the body of the gallbladder (Fig. 5.10 a–e).

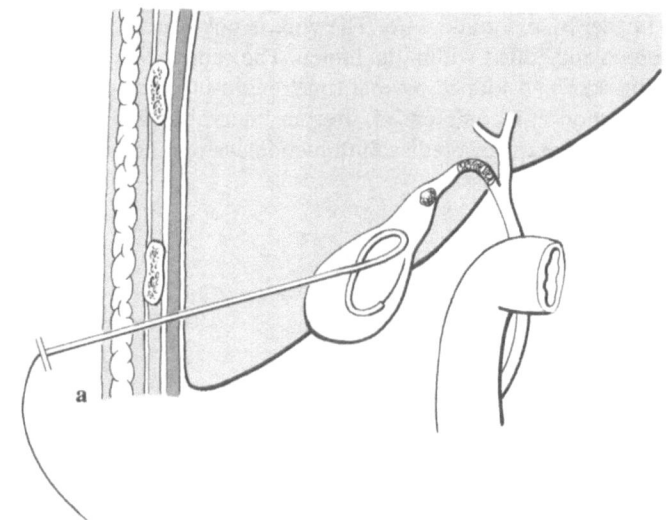

Fig. 5. 10 a–e. Method of retrieving a stone from the neck of the gallbladder using a guide wire. **a** A guide wire is reintroduced into the gallbladder via the lysis catheter. **b** A loop of the catheter-covered wire is pushed into the neck of the gallbladder to entrap the stone. **c** The catheter and wire are partly withdrawn with the stone into the fundus of the gallbladder

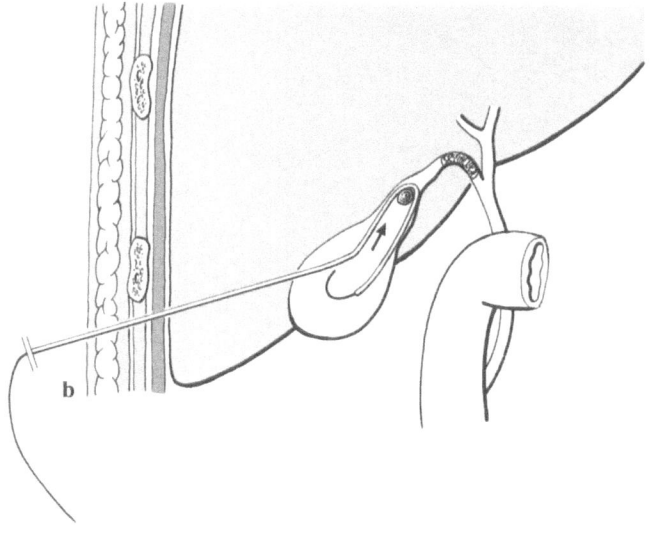

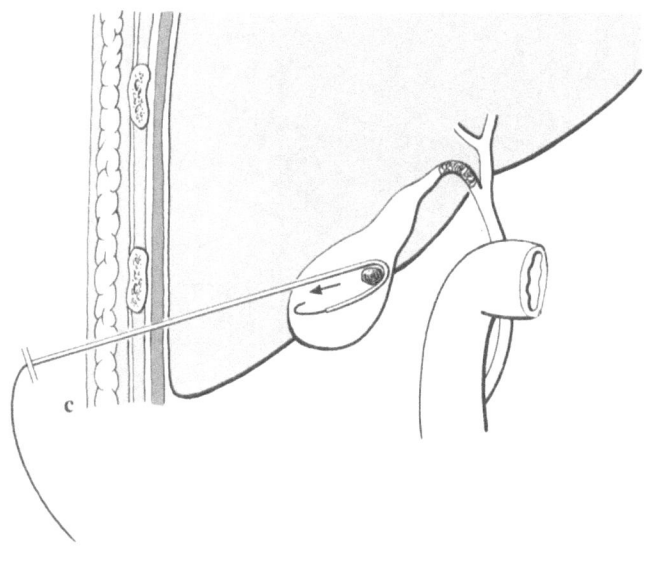

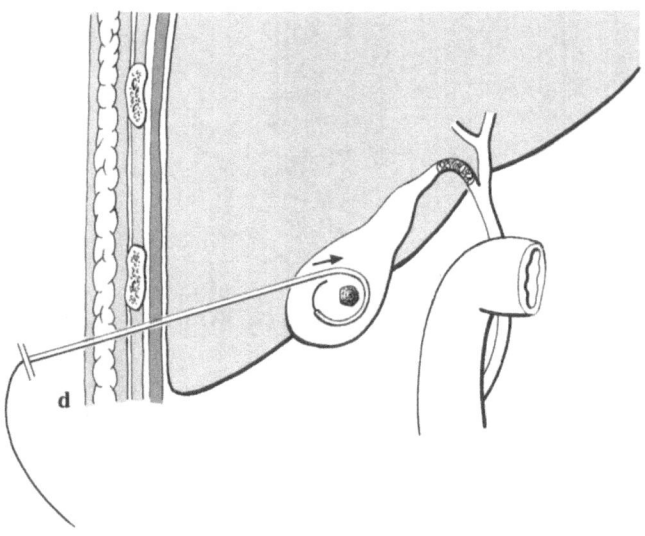

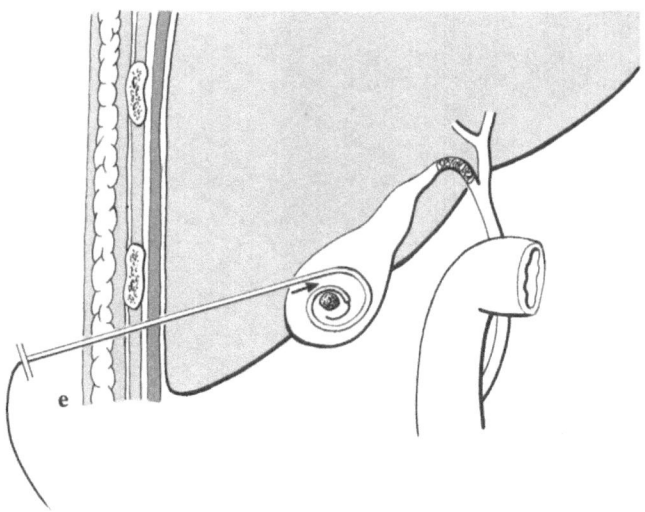

Fig. 5.10 d, e. The catheter is looped around the stone

Removal of the Transhepatic Catheter from the Gallbladder

The transhepatic catheter is removed in the Radiology Department on the fluo-roscopy table under sterile conditions with analgesia. A guide wire is introduced into the gallbladder through the pigtail catheter. The catheter is freed at the skin and it is slowly withdrawn over the wire; the wire tip is left within the lumen. The guide wire is used to uncoil the catheter, and this prevents the catheter loops from adhering to each other; this would make a much larger hole in the wall of the gall-bladder and increase the risk of bile leakage.

The final cholecystocholangiogram made before removal of the catheter should demonstrate clearly the cystic duct and the bile ducts down to the duodenum to show that no stone fragments have passed from the gallbladder into the common bile duct during stone dissolution. When this study is completed, as much contrast medium as possible is aspirated from the gallbladder before removal of the catheter, to minimise any leakage (Fig. 5.11 a, b).

Finally, the hole in the liver capsule is plugged with Gelfoam [2]. This is done by inserting a small catheter over the guide wire for a distance of 4–5 cm from the

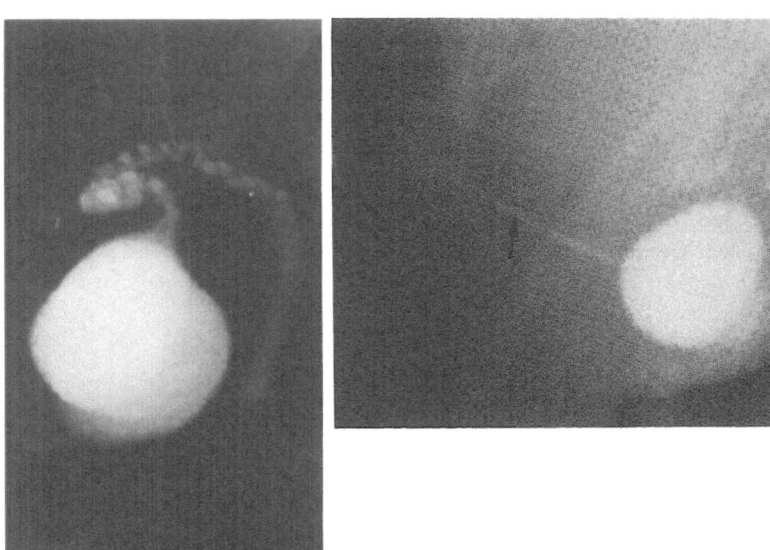

a

b

Fig. 5.11. a Final percutaneous contrast examination of the gallbladder after stone lysis. **b** The cholecystostomy catheter has been removed and a track of contrast medium is seen traversing the liver from gallbladder to the liver capsule (*arrow*). Flow of contrast medium stopped within 3 min. Occluding the track with Gelfoam prevents any contrast or bile from spilling. The gallbladder should be emptied of contrast medium and bile before the catheter is removed

skin into the liver. The wire is removed and compressed Gelfoam strips are inserted down the catheter with a wire as the short the catheter is removed.

The patient is kept in hospital overnight while the vital signs are monitored. The following morning, the gallbladder is examined by ultrasound and this may show some debris. If all stone material has been removed this debris shows no acoustic shadowing on ultrasound examination. Most patients are symptom free at this stage; some experience mild upper abdominal pain for 24 h. None of our patients have required readmission to hospital for any reason related to MTBE dissolution therapy. Only patients who are symptom free are permitted to leave the hospital. At 3 months and at 6 months an ultrasound examination of the gallbladder is performed to look for stone recurrence.

References

1. Allen MJ, Borody TJ, Bugliosi TF, May GR, La Russo NF, Thistle JL (1985) Rapid dissolution of gallstones with methyl tert butyl ether. N Engl J Med 312:217–220
2. Bender CE, Williams HJ (1988) Technical aspects of percutaneous gallstone dissolution. Semin Intervent Radiol 5:186–194
3. Hellstern A, Leuschner M, Fisher H, Lazarovici D, Gullutuna S, Kurtz W, Leuschner U (1988) Percutantranshepatische Lyse von Gallenblasensteinen mit Methyl-tert-butyläther. Dtsch Med Wochenschr 113:506–510
4. Ponchon T, Baround J, Pujol B, Vallette PJ, Perrot D (1988) Renal failure during dissolution of gallstones with methyl tert butyl ether. Lancet 2:276–277
5. Thistle JL, May GR, Bender CE, Williams HJ et al. (1989) Dissolution of cholesterol gallbladder stones by methyl tert butyl ether administered by percutaneous transhepatic catheter. N Engl J Med 320:633–639
6. Zakko SF, Hofmann AF, Schteingart C, van Sonnenberg E, Wheeler HO (1987) Percutaneous gallbladder stone dissolution using a microprocessor-assisted solvent transfer (MAST) system. Gastroenterology 92:1794 (abstract)

CHAPTER 6

Percutaneous Cholecystostomy for Biliary Drainage

Acute Gallbladder Disease

Percutaneous cholecystostomy may be used to drain the inflammed gallbladder in acute cholecystitis with or without gallstones. The technique may also be used for emergency treatment of mucocoele of empyema of the gallbladder. The patient who is unfit for surgery because of advanced age, cardiac failure, pulmonary disease, renal failure, liver failure, severe sepsis or immunosuppression benefits most from percutaneous gallbladder drainage. Our experience is that the patient with acute gallbladder disease who is fit for surgery should have surgical cholecystectomy as soon as the diagnosis is established.

Sectional imaging is essential for successful emergency gallbladder drainage. Ultrasound is essential to localise the gallbladder in the emergency situation, and CT scanning is valuable in selecting the best site for percutaneous gallbladder puncture in order to avoid intervening intestine. A transhepatic route to the gallbladder is safest.

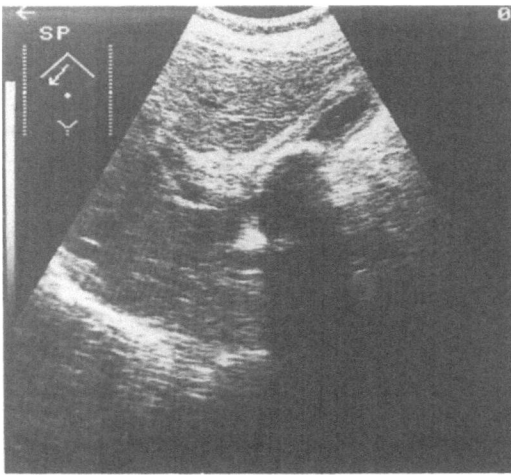

Fig. 6.1. Ultrasound of the gallbladder in acute cholecystitis showing a stone in the neck of a small, thick-walled gallbladder. The organ is too small for percutaneous drainage

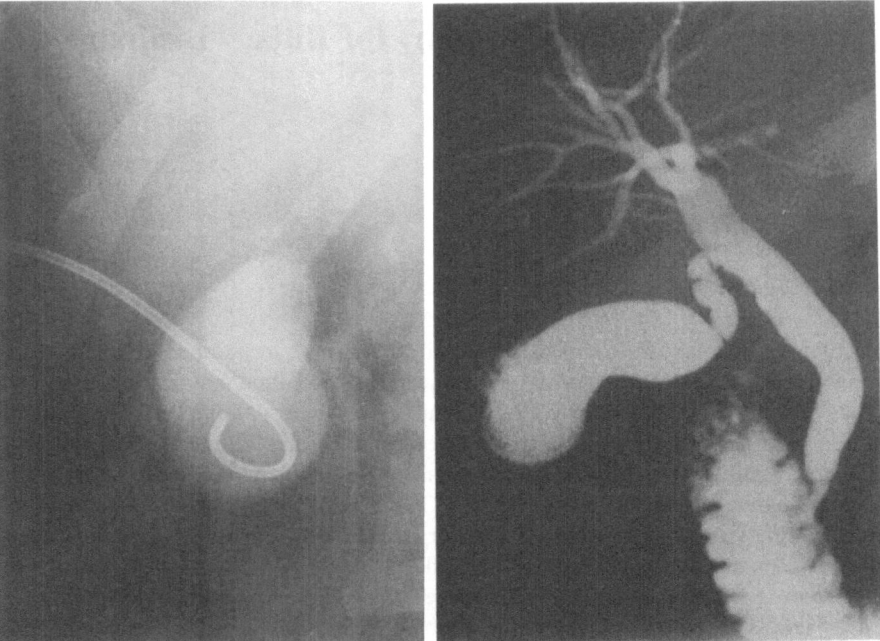

a   b

Fig. 6.2. a Cholangiogram showing "single-stab" catheter insertion in calculous cholecystitis. Bile has been removed and dilute contrast medium introduced into the gallbladder at
24 h. The cystic duct is occluded. Patient was a 52-year-old woman with right upper quadrant pain and vomiting and with a tender, nonpalpable gallbladder. The WBC was
14 000 mm^3. **b** Repeat cholangiogram at 7 days via the cholecystostomy tube showed no
calculi, a patent cystic duct and unobstructed biliary ducts

We have used both the Seldinger technique and the direct-catheter-over-needle
method to puncture the inflammed gallbladder using a transhepatic route (Fig.
6.2 a, b). Because the inflammed gallbladder wall is easily traumatised, the least
manipulation within the organ in the acute situation is preferred (Fig. 6.3); hence,
a single puncture of the gallbladder with a catheter over a needle is best.

The examination is preferably performed in the Radiology Unit on a fluoroscopic table with high-resolution ultrasound control of the site of gallbladder
puncture. Fluoroscopy is then used to confirm the location of the catheter within
the gallbladder. Bile is aspirated from the organ for culture, and dilute contrast
medium is carefully injected to confirm the catheter location but not to opacify the
cystic duct or bile ducts; this may be undertaken after 24–48 h of drainage.

Drainage of a mucocoele or empyema of the gallbladder is easier to perform
because of the distended gallbladder. When the gallbladder is visible or palpable
anteriorly below the liver the anterior subcostal route may be used.

With an enlarged gallbladder it is better to coil several loops of catheter within
the organ to allow for gallbladder shrinkage. It may also be necessary to penetrate

the wall of the organ with a dilator over a guide wire before inserting the drainage catheter in order to avoid buckling of the catheter at the gallbladder wall, with possible loss of the organ.

Alternatively, a rigid Lunderquist wire may be used to insert the catheter into the gallbladder lumen; it should be kept in mind that this wire must be fixed externally by an assistant during catheter insertion. Following successful percutaneous cholecystostomy the catheter is attached to a closed drainage system.

The causal lesion in mucocoele or empyema is often a calculus. This may fall back into the gallbladder when the organ is drained. Following 24–48 h of drainage the gallbladder is markedly reduced in size, and at this stage transcatheter cholecystocholangiography may be performed to assess the cause of the mucocoele and the patency of the cystic duct and the extrahepatic bile ducts. Manipulation within the gallbladder should not be undertaken for at least 1 week after initial gallbladder drainage. At this time a stone in the neck of the gallbladder may be retrieved into the gallbladder using a loop of guide wire. A stone in the cystic duct may be removed with a dormia basket introduced via the drainage catheter.

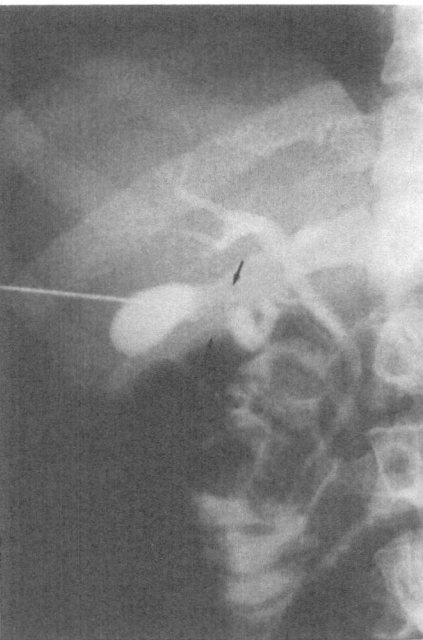

Fig. 6.3. Needle/catheter introduced with great difficulty into a thick-walled gallbladder demonstrated a large solitary stone (*arrows*). Introduction of a guide wire for catheterisation failed, as the wire could not be coiled in the small area of gallbladder below the stone. It caused a large perforation in the friable gallbladder wall which required cholecystectomy

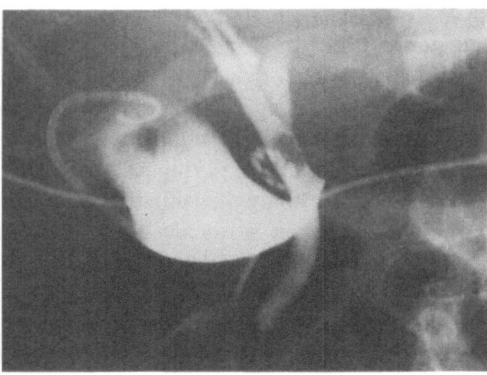

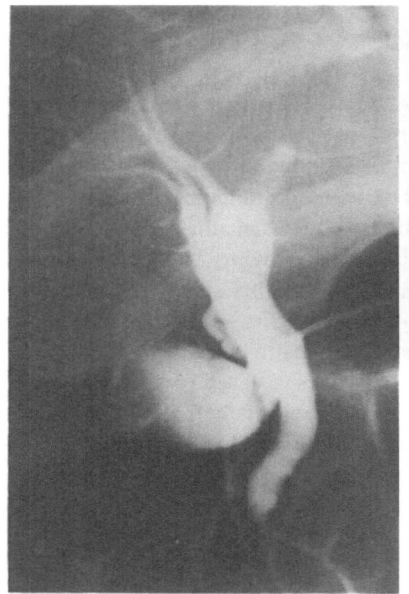

a

Fig. 6.4 a, b. A 68-year-old woman with ascending cholangitis was treated by endoscopic insertion of a nasobiliary catheter. Cholangiography via the catheter demonstrated large gallstones and a common duct stone (**a**). Since pus was recovered from the bile ducts suppurative cholecystitis was suspected, and using a percutaneous transhepatic route the gallbladder was catheterised and a 9-French pigtail catheter was coiled within the gallbladder for drainage. (**b**). The gallstones were dissolved using MTBE after endoscopic removal of the bile duct stone and recovery from the cholangitis

Extrahepatic Biliary Obstruction

Percutaneous cholecystostomy for drainage in cases of extrahepatic biliary obstruction is of value only when the obstruction lies below the junction of the cystic and common hepatic ducts. We have used the technique to drain the biliary tract when endoscopic and transhepatic drainage have failed or when the patient was too ill to undergo these procedures. It is a palliative procedure in the very ill patient. We have also used the technique in gross biliary sepsis with suppurative ascending cholangitis where cholelithiasis was present with multiple gallstones (Fig. 6.4).

Percutaneous cholecystostomy for drainage is performed using a transhepatic approach to the gallbladder, which is often opacified following diagnostic transhepatic or endoscopic cholangiography. Using adequate sedation, analgesia and local anaesthesia and a sterile technique, a catheter needle is introduced transhepatically into the upper third of the body of the gallbladder. The needle is removed and replaced by a semi-stiff guide wire which is looped in the gallbladder. A dilator is introduced over the guide wire into the gallbladder. The dilator is removed and replaced by a 5-French pigtail catheter with multiple side holes in the loop. At least two loops of the catheter are coiled in the gallbladder. The catheter is fixed to the skin of the axilla and attached to a closed drainage system.

CHAPTER 7

Percutaneous Cholecystostomy for Gallstone Removal and Access to the Bile Ducts

Indications

Percutaneous cholecystostomy for the removal of gallstones is used as an alternative to cholecystectomy in patients with calcified gallstones. The advantage of the technique is that all gallstones are removed immediately, regardless of composition, size or number of calculi [1–3]. It may also be used to complete the process of stone removal immediately after ECSWL of gallstones and to prevent stone fragments from passing into the bile ducts.

Percutaneous cholecystostomy and minilaparotomy cholecystostomy have been used to gain access to the bile ducts for stone removal. This method is seldom necessary when expert endoscopic experience is available.

Preparation of the Patient and Gallbladder Assessment

We prefer that the patient for percutaneous cholecystolithotomy have a normally functioning gallbladder with a normal wall thickness, as determined by computed tomography and ultrasonography. Normal function, judged on the basis of an opacified gallbladder at oral cholecystography, is not necessary for successful stone removal, but in the absence of gallbladder function a better alternative treatment for gallstones is surgical cholecystectomy. The procedure is contraindicated in the presence of a small contracted gallbladder or a calcified gallbladder. Acute cholecystitis is also a contraindication. A thickened gallbladder wall makes puncture of the organ and dilatation of a track to the gallbladder lumen much more difficult. Loss of the track during puncture or dilatation requires surgery, since the diseased gallbladder wall cannot contract to stop the leakage of bile.

Ultrasound examination and CT are used to study the relationship of the gallbladder to the liver and the colon. CT sagittal reconstructions help to evaluate puncture site, angle of the needle and distance of the puncture site from the gallbladder. Gallstones with a high CT number or seen as calcified on a plain film of the abdomen are suitable for this form of treatment. We prefer to use sedation and analgesia with local anaesthesia for all applications of percutaneous cholecystostomy, including percutaneous lithotomy. The patient who is unfit for general anaesthesia because of cardiac, respiratory or other diseases may be treated by this method of gallstone removal. We believe, however, that patients who are fit for anaesthesia should have a surgical cholecystectomy for calcified gallstones.

The patient is admitted to hospital on the evening before the procedure Gallbladder and gallstone assessments are carried out prior to admission. A coagulation screen excludes any coagulation disorder. The contraindications listed in Chap. 2 are strictly enforced.

The procedure is performed in the fasting patient, and hydration is maintained with i.v. fluids. The procedure is performed in the Radiology Department using a standard undercouch fluoroscopic tilting table. Preprocedure preparations include intravenous antibiotics, sedation and analgesia.

The patient is positioned supine on the fluoroscopy table. Adequate covering of the patient is necessary to maintain body heat during the lithotripsy procedure. With a combination of CT images, fluoroscopy and lateral positioning of the ultrasound probe, a right subcostal site is chosen for gallbladder puncture and the skin site is marked. The abdomen is covered with waterproof surgical sheets which also protect the X-ray table from endoscopic irrigation fluid. The latter is drained into a suitable container to prevent electrical hazards.

Technique of Catheterisation [2–4] (Fig. 7.1 a–g)

Using a sterile technique, the skin and abdominal wall down to the peritoneum over the gallbladder fundus are infiltrated with local anaesthetic. A crosswise incision is made with a scalpel, and a track is made to the peritoneum using mosquito forceps. A catheter/needle[1] is inserted into the fundus of the gallbladder with a stabbing motion (Fig. 7.1 a). The needle is removed, and if the catheter lies within the lumen, bile drips from the catheter (Fig. 7.1 b). A guide wire is inserted into the gallbladder and coiled in the lumen. A 5-French pigtail catheter is inserted over the wire and coiled in the gallbladder. The wire is now removed (Fig. 7.1 c). The bile is aspirated from the gallbladder and contrast medium is injected to outline the gallstones, the cystic duct and the common bile duct. The gallbladder is irrigated with saline until the return is clear of bile. A small amount of contrast medium is now injected to outline the gallbladder. The gallbladder volume is kept as small as possible by aspiration after the organ is irrigated. At this stage, the pigtail catheter is removed over a guide wire and replaced by a 5-French dilator. This dilator is used to attempt to insert a special hydrophilic, coated guide wire (Amlpatz Torque[1] Teflon coated) into the cystic duct and common bile duct and duodenum (Fig. 7.1 d). If this is achieved it greatly increases stability of the guide wire during dilator insertion. A steerable catheter may also be used to direct the wire to the neck of the gallbladder and into the cystic duct.

---

[1] Meditech, USA.

If the wire fails to enter the cystic duct it is coiled in the gallbladder. At this stage, a 5- or 6-French dilator is inserted over the wire. This is replaced by either a balloon dilator or the first of a set of coaxial dilators (Fig. 7.1 f). In one step, the Olbert balloon dilator produces a track to the gallbladder of 1 cm in diameter. A working sheath may be backloaded on the balloon catheter with a dilator. The balloon is deflated and the dilator is inserted over it, followed by the working sheath. Alternatively, a series of coaxial dilators are inserted into the gallbladder until the track is dilated to 18 French, and a Teflon sheath of this size is inserted into the gallbladder lumen (Fig. 7.1 g).

During dilator insertion the dilators should always be pointed towards the patients head. They are always held in place manually, close to the skin, an acute angle being maintained with the skin of the abdominal wall. At this stage we decide whether to perform a one-stage stone-removal procedure or to continue the procedure at a later date. The decision is based on the ease of gallbladder catheterisation, the size and number of calculi present, the state of the gallbladder wall (i.e. is the wall diseased or not?), whether it was possible to insert a guide wire into the cystic duct and common bile duct and whether the patient was classified fit for general anaesthesia at preprocedure assessment. If it is decided to delay stone removal, a 14-French Foley catheter is inserted down the 18-French Teflon sheath. it is inflated *before the sheath is removed*, and the patient

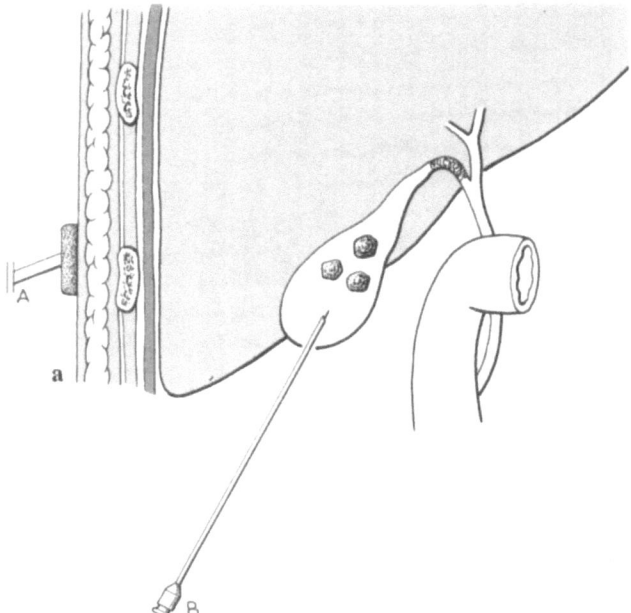

Fig. 7.1 a–g. Percutaneous subcostal cholecystostomy for cholecystolithotomy. **a** Subcostal puncture of the fundus of the gallbladder with a catheter/needle: *A*, ultrasound probe; *B*, 19 SWG catheter/needle

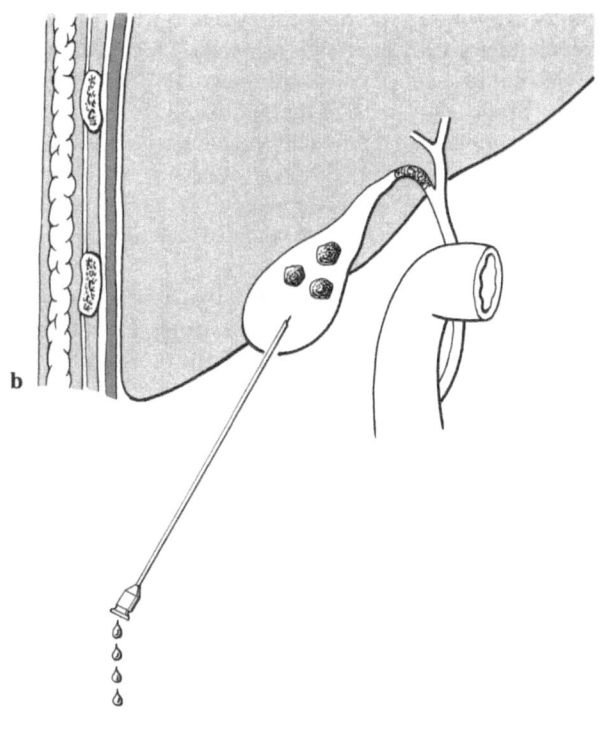

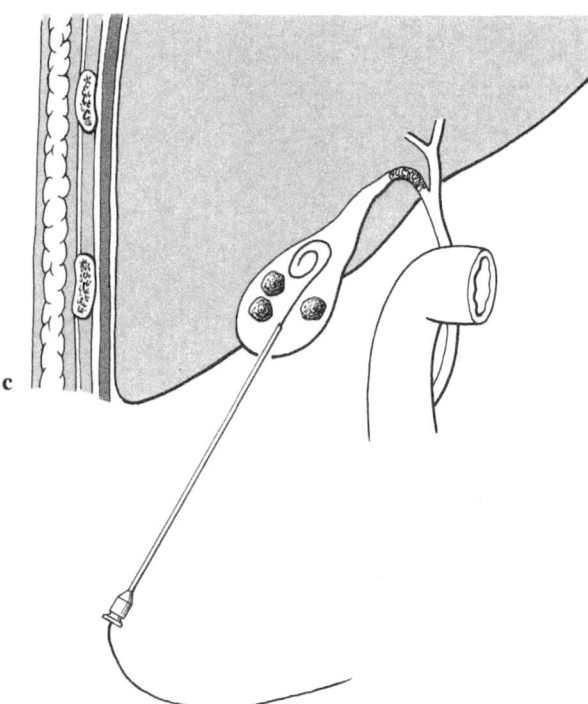

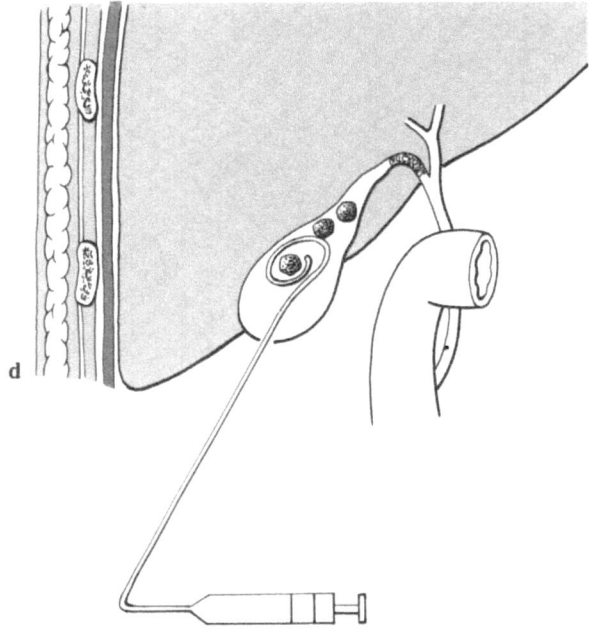

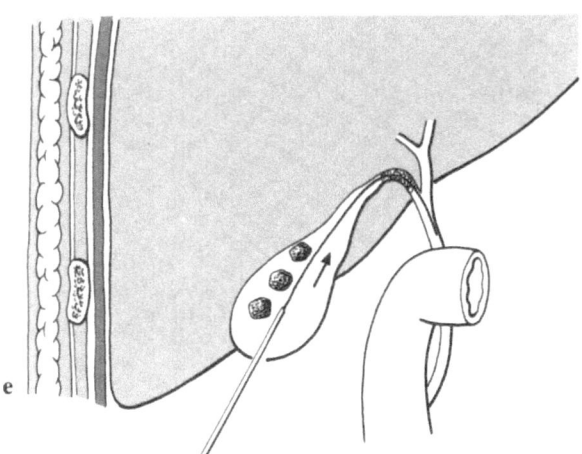

Fig. 7.1. b Black bile drains from the catheter when the catheter lies in the gallbladder lumen. **c** Guide wire is coiled within the gallbladder. **d** 5-French pigtail catheter is inserted over the wire into the gallbladder for bile removal and irrigation until the gallbladder is bile free. **e** Guide wire is inserted via the straightened pigtail catheter into the cystic duct and common bile duct

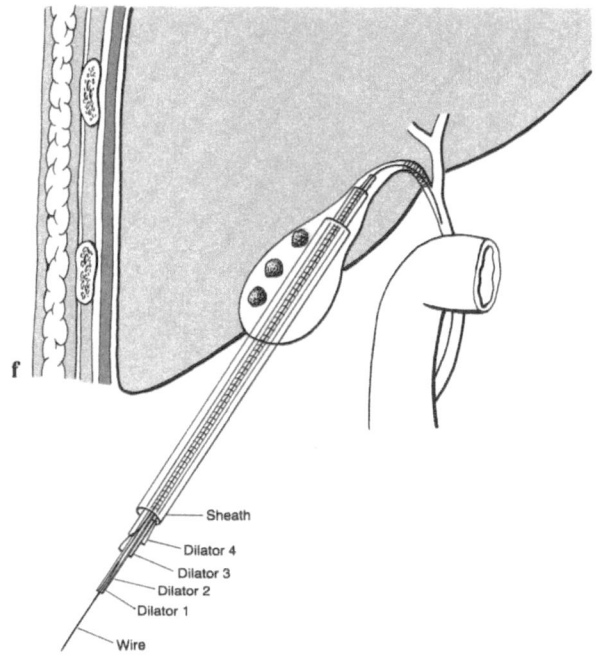

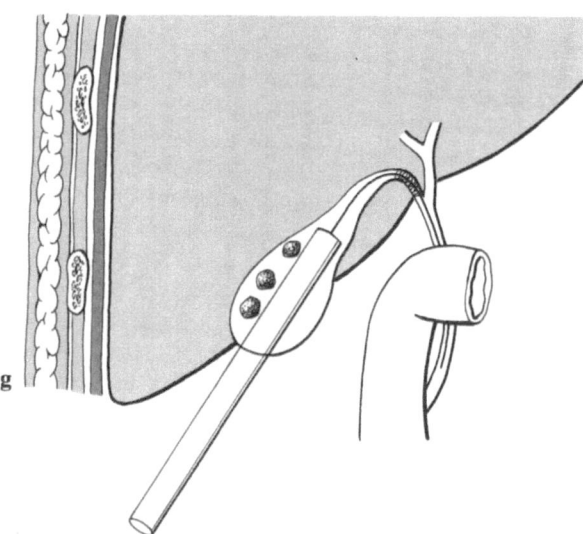

Fig. 7.1.f A series of coaxial dilators are inserted into the gallbladder and a working sheath is inserted over the largest dilator. **g** The dilators are removed and the working sheath is held manually within the gallbladder

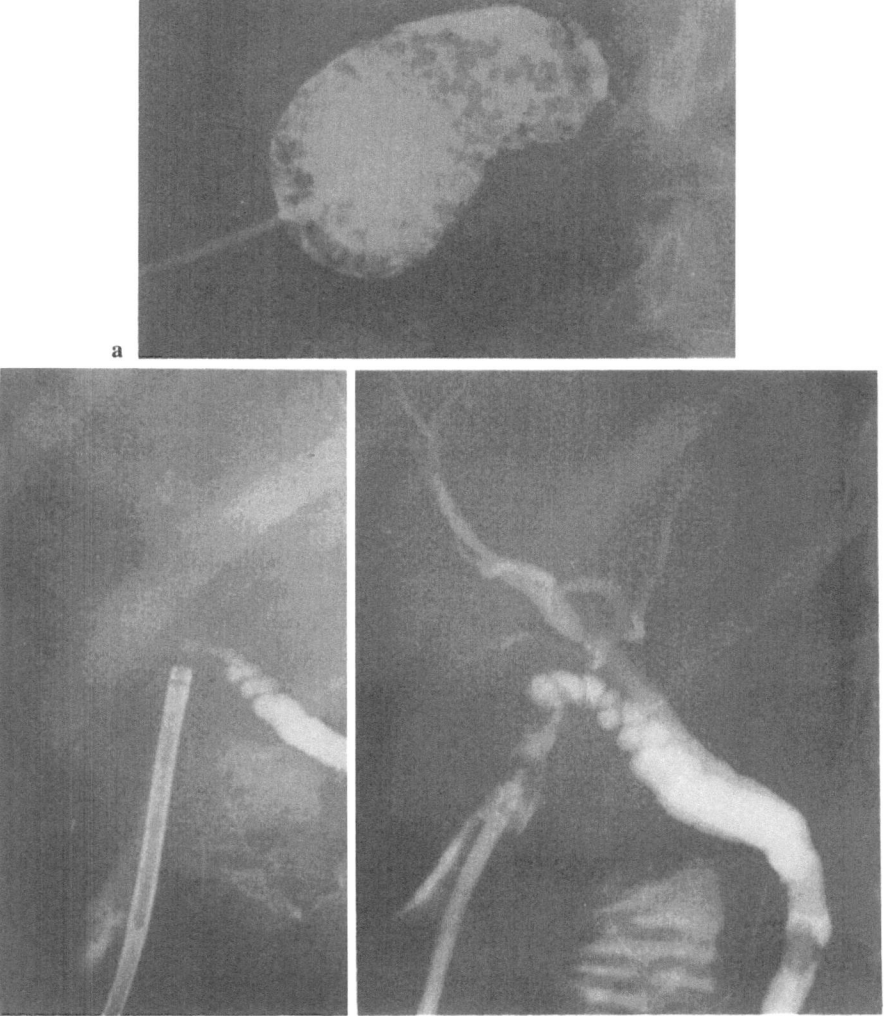

Fig. 7.2 a–f. A 67-year-old man with a history of two cerebrovascular accidents and multiple gallbladder stones with CT numbers of 180+ was referred for nonoperative stone removal. Following percutaneous puncture of the fundus of the gallbladder, a 5-French pigtail catheter was inserted with difficulty into the gallbladder over a Lunderquist wire. Only one loop of catheter could be placed in the gallbladder (**a**). Attempts at inserting a guide wire into the cystic duct failed at this stage. One loop of a semi-stiff guide wire was coiled in the gallbladder and, after insertion of a 5-French dilator over the wire, a track was dilated to 18 French with biliary coaxial dilators. Next an 18-French sheath was inserted into the gallbladder. Many small calculi were removed by a combination of suction, irrigation with saline and basket removal (**b**). A Foley catheter was inserted into the gallbladder and a cholecystocholangiogram performed (**c**). This demonstrated a solitary stone low down in a long cystic duct

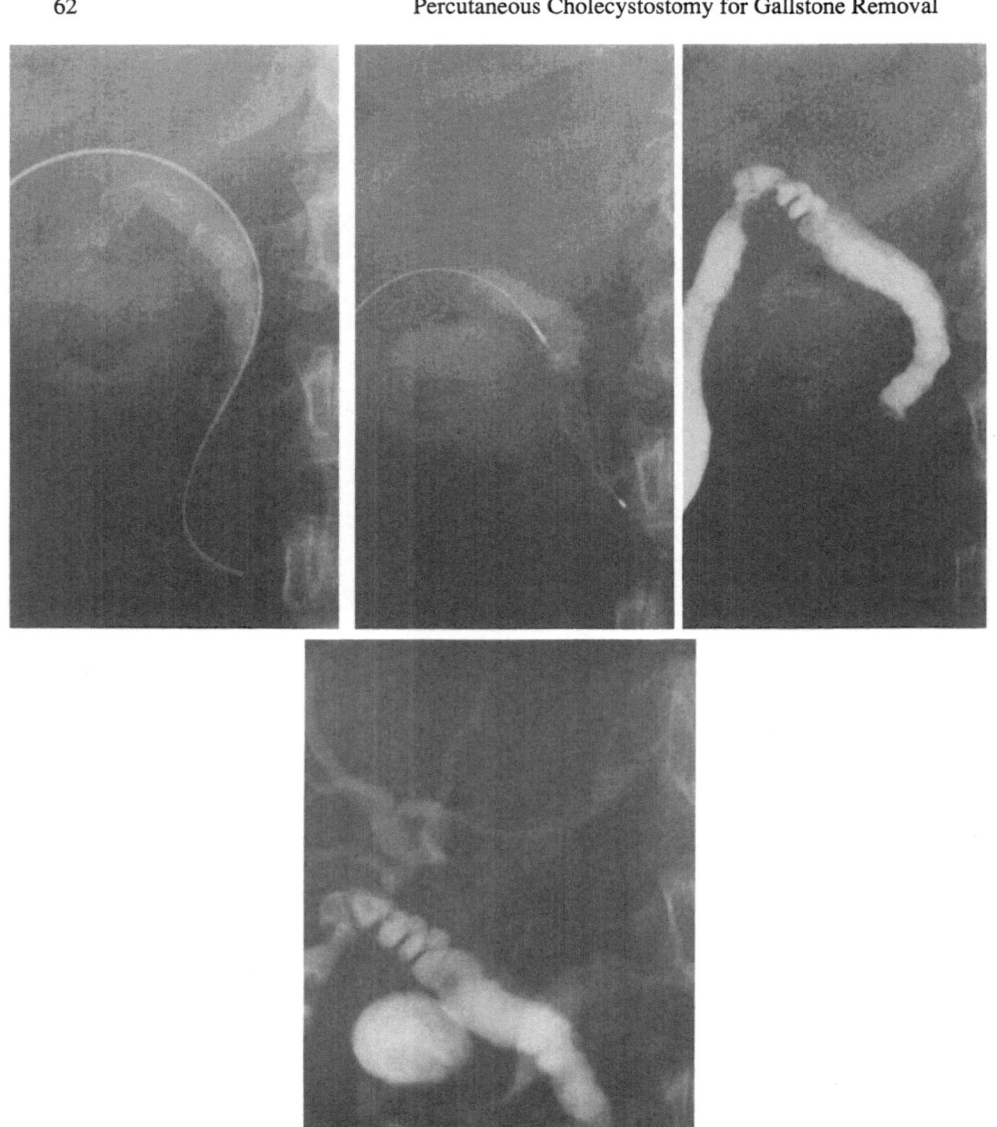

d   e

f

returns for procedure completion in 3–7 days. The patient may go home after 24 h and return at the appointed time for stone removal. After 3–7 days the fundus of the gallbladder is adherent to the abdominal wall and loss of the gallbladder is unlikely. The Foley catheter is removed over a guide wire and the cholecystostomy track is now dilated to 25 French. A working sheath is inserted over the final dilator into the gallbladder.

The 25-French sheath allows easy access to the gallbladder. If the stones are small they are removed by irrigation, suction, grasping forceps or a dormia wire basket (Fig. 7.2).

Larger stones require fragmentation by electrohydraulic lithotripsy using a 3-French electrode and direct vision with a flexible choledochoscope. Great care is taken to avoid contact with the wall of the gallbladder. Most stones are fragmented by two to four shocks, although additional shocks are necessary to fragment larger stones. During lithotripsy, irrigation with N/6 saline allows good conduction of shock waves. After stone removal the gallbladder is inspected for remaining stones. When the gallbladder is visibly free of stone debris, a 14-French Foley catheter is inserted down the sheath and inflated *before the sheath is removed.* The catheter is connected to a closed biliary drainage bag and the patient is returned to the ward.

Fig. 7.2 d–f. After 24 h the patient was returned for removal of the cystic duct stone. This was carried out by inserting a guide wire down the duct, followed by a dormia basket, and withdrawing the calculus into the gallbladder (**d** and **e**). A repeat cholangiogram (**f**) showed the duct system and gallbladder to be free of gallstones. Two days later, the gallbladder and bile were checked by cholecystocholangiography for gallstones; the gallbladder was emptied and the Foley catheter was removed. The patient was discharged 1 day later. Nine months later he remains well and the gallbladder is free of gallstones

Postprocedure Management

After successful gallstone removal, care of the biliary drainage bag is essential. Analgesia is given as required. After 24 h a contrast study is made of the gallbladder and if it, the cystic duct and bile ducts are stone free the gallbladder is emptied of contrast medium and bile and the catheter is removed. The patient is discharged 24 h later.

Complications

Percutaneous track dilatation to the gallbladder is a difficult procedure. The major disaster during this procedure is *loss of the gallbladder*. This can be prevented by inserting a guide wire down the cystic duct into the common bile duct and duodenum. Use of a special hydrophilic, coated guide wire assists cystic duct cannulation. We have also used an 8-French steerable catheter to direct the wire into the neck of the gallbladder and help with cystic duct catheterisation. The Teflon coaxial dilators are easier to insert into the gallbladder than replacement dilators, and with the former there is less risk of losing the gallbladder. Coaxial metal dilators may also be used.

The Olbert balloon dilator system allows for one-step dilatation of the track and also reduces the risk of loss of the gallbladder. During gallbladder irrigation a *stone fragment may pass into the cystic duct or common bile duct*. This may be prevented by having the guide wire within the cystic duct-common bile duct system.

When a stone fragment passes into the cystic duct it may be retrieved into the gallbladder using a dormia basket (Fig. 7.2 d). A stone fragment in the common bile duct requires removal by endoscopic sphincterotomy and basket extraction.

Perforation of the gallbladder may occur during electrohydraulic lithotripsy. Catheter drainage of the gallbladder when this occurs may prevent bile leakage and obviate the need for emergency cholecystectomy. Successful stone removal requires the services of a skilled interventional radiologist, an expert endoscopist and a skilled endourologist.

References

1. Bender CE, Le Roy AJ, Segura JW, van Heeden A, Hughes RW, Thistle JL (1989) Percutaneous cholecystolithotomy. Paper read at Society of Biliary Radiology meeting, November 29, Chicago
2. Hruby W, Stackl W, Urban M, Armbruster C, Marburger M (1989) Percutaneous endoscopic cholecystolithotripsy. Work in progress. Radiology 173:477–479
3. Kellet MJ, Wickham JEA, Russell RCG (1988) Percutaneous cholecystolithotomy. Br Med J 296:453–455
4. Kerlan RK, LaBerge JM, Ring EJ (1985) Percutaneous cholecystolithotomy: preliminary experience. Radiology 157:653–656
5. Cope C, Burke DR, Meranze SG (1990) Percutaneous extraction of gallstones in 20 patients. Radiology 176:19–24
6. Akiyama H, Okazaki T, Tahashima I et al. (1990) Percutaneous treatments for biliary disease. Radiology 176:25–30

J. Albores-Saavedra, University of Texas, Dallas, TX;
D. E. Henson, Bethesda, MD;
L. H. Sobin, Washingon, D. C.

Histological Typing of Tumours of the Gallbladder and Extrahepatic Bile Ducts

In collaboration with pathologists in 5 countries

2nd ed. 1990. Approx. 100 pp. 90 figs. (WHO – International Histological Classification of Tumours) Softcover DM 68,–
ISBN 3-540-52838-5

(Originally published by the WHO in No. 20 in the International Histological Classification of Tumours series)

The second edition of **Histological Typing of Tumours of the Gallbladder and Extrahepatic Bile Ducts** is more extensive and detailed than the previous edition. It includes a detailed histological classification of tumours and tumour-like lesions of the gallbladder and extrahepatic bile ducts and also describes the salient histological features. The usefulness of new techniques such as immunohistochemistry is emphasized. This histological classification will facilitate pathologic, therapeutic and epidemiologic comparisons.

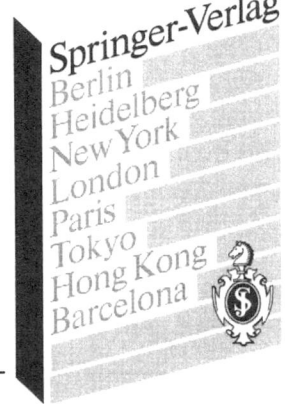

Springer-Verlag
Berlin
Heidelberg
New York
London
Paris
Tokyo
Hong Kong
Barcelona

B. Deixonne, Nîmes; **F.-M. Lopez,** University of Montpellier-Nîmes (Eds.)

Operative Ultrasonography

During Hepatobiliary and Pancreatic Surgery

With the Collaboration of M. Dauzat, M. Makuuchi, J. Mouroux, A. Pissas and B. Sigel

Foreword by H. Baumel

Translated by J. Simon

1988. XII, 135 pp. 124 figs. Hardcover DM 148,–
ISBN 3-540-17630-6

This book deals with the use of ultrasound during hepatobiliary and pancreatic surgery. This ultrasound technique represents one of the best means of perioperative exploration in this field. The work thus aims to provide surgeons with a precise description of ultrasonography including the theoretical as well as the practical bases for its application. Furthermore, three different chapters deal with ultrasonography of the liver, biliary ducts and pancreas. Each chapter begins by reviewing surgical anatomy, exploration methodology and echographic semiology, and then mentions specific problems of the organs.

Hepatobiliary and pancreatic surgery is being increasingly absorbed into the framework of general and digestive surgery. Here perioperative ultrasonography proves to be indispensible, not only for the confirmation or assessment of diagnosis, but also for establishing the best therapeutic strategy. It is a useful complement to the surgeon's eye and hand.

Prices are subject to change without notice.

Springer-Verlag
Berlin
Heidelberg
New York
London
Paris
Tokyo
Hong Kong
Barcelona